W0115401

13081

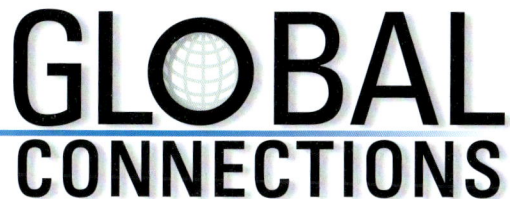

GLOBAL CONNECTIONS

PANDEMICS AND GLOBAL HEALTH

GLOBAL CONNECTIONS

America's Role in a Changing World
Changing Climates
The Changing Global Economy
Environment and Natural Resources
Feeding a Hungry World
The Human Population
Human Rights
One World or Many?
Pandemics and Global Health
Terrorism and Security

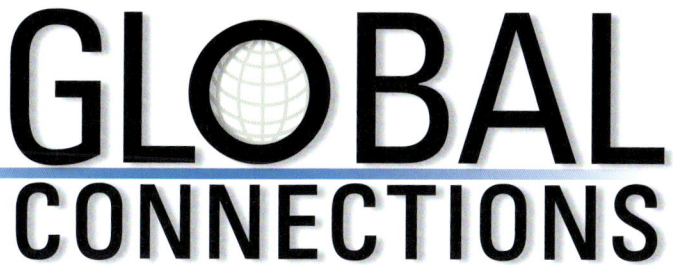

GLOBAL CONNECTIONS

PANDEMICS AND GLOBAL HEALTH

JOSEPH R. OPPONG
SERIES EDITOR: CHARLES F. GRITZNER

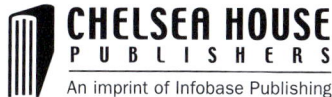

CHELSEA HOUSE
PUBLISHERS
An imprint of Infobase Publishing

Chelsea House
An imprint of Infobase Publishing
132 West 31st Street
New York, NY 10001

Library of Congress Cataloging-in-Publication Data
Oppong, Joseph R.
 Pandemics and global health / by Joseph R. Oppong.
    p. cm. — (Global Connections)
 Includes bibliographical references and index.
 ISBN 978-1-60413-285-4 (hardcover)
 1. World health. 2. Public health—International cooperation. I. Title.
II. Series.

 RA441.O67 2010
 362.1—dc22   2009033605

Chelsea House books are available at special discounts when purchased in bulk quantities for businesses, associations, institutions, or sales promotions. Please call our Special Sales Department in New York at (212) 967-8800 or (800) 322-8755.

You can find Chelsea House on the World Wide Web
at http://www.chelseahouse.com

Text design by Annie O'Donnell
Cover design by Takeshi Takahashi
Composition by EJB Publishing Services
Cover printed by Bang Printing, Brainerd, MN
Book printed and bound by Bang Printing, Brainerd, MN
Date printed: May 2010
Printed in the United States of America

10 9 8 7 6 5 4 3 2 1

This book is printed on acid-free paper.

All links and Web addresses were checked and verified to be correct at the time of publication. Because of the dynamic nature of the Web, some addresses and links may have changed since publication and may no longer be valid.

CONTENTS

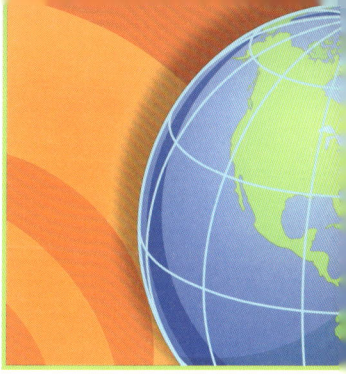

Introduction: A Global Community   7

1   Introduction to Global Health Issues   9

2   Health Geography and Global Health   18

3   Pandemics, Epidemics, and Endemics   29

4   HIV/AIDS   39

5   Tuberculosis   53

6   Polio   62

7   The Coming Pandemics?   79

8   Emerging and Reemerging Pandemics   96

Glossary   107

Bibliography   110

Further Resources   111

Picture Credits   113

Index   114

About the Author and Editor   119

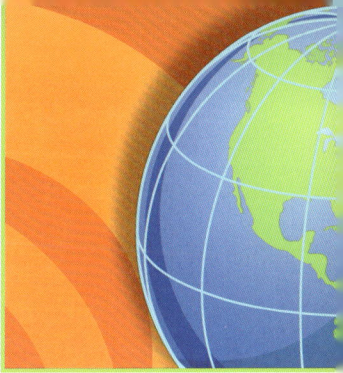

INTRODUCTION

A GLOBAL COMMUNITY

Globalization is the process of coming together as a closely connected global community. It began thousands of years ago, when tribal groups and small hunting parties wandered from place to place. The process accelerated following Columbus's epic voyage more than five centuries ago. Europeans—an estimated 50 million of them—spread out to occupy lands throughout the world. This migration transformed the distribution of the world's peoples and their cultures forever. In the United States and Canada, for example, most people speak a West European language. Most practice a religious faith with roots in the ancient Middle East and eat foods originating in Asia.

Today, we are citizens of a closely interwoven global community. Events occurring half a world away can be watched and experienced, often as they happen, in our own homes. People, materials, and even diseases can be transported from continent to continent in a single day, thanks to jet planes. Electronic communications make possible the instantaneous exchange of information by phone, e-mail, or other means with friends or business associates almost anywhere in the world. Trade and commerce, perhaps more so than any other aspect of our daily lives, amply illustrate the importance of global linkages. How many things in your home (including your clothing) are of international origin? What foods and beverages have you consumed today that came from other lands? Could Northern America's economy survive without foreign oil, iron ore, copper, or other vital resources?

The GLOBAL CONNECTIONS series is designed to help you realize how closely people and places are tied to one another within the expanding global community. Each book introduces you to political, economic, environmental, social, medical, and other timely issues, problems, and prospects. The authors and editors hope you enjoy and learn from these books. May they hand you a passport to intellectual travels throughout our fascinating, complex, and increasingly "intradependent" world!

—Charles F. Gritzner
Series Editor

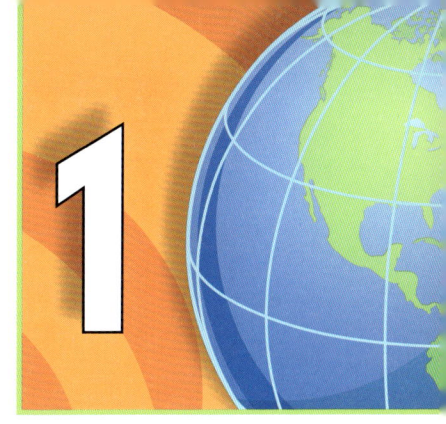

INTRODUCTION TO GLOBAL HEALTH ISSUES

Never before has the threat of global pandemic diseases been so high. New diseases are emerging at record rates. They cross borders easily and rapidly. Diseases that previously were considered controlled have returned as threats. Some of them are even more deadly than before. Previously unknown diseases have become common. Rising drug resistance has made many trusted wonder drugs ineffective. New health threats keep emerging with the changing global climate. As a result, fatal communicable diseases threaten all humans. No country can fully protect its citizens by isolating them or through traditional border controls.

Can we prevent another major global disease outbreak? Why do diseases emerge in certain places and not in others? How do diseases spread between places? Does human risk of disease vary with place of residence? How about income and wealth? Do diseases affect mostly poor people or do economics not matter? Why are some countries severely affected by HIV/AIDS while others are not? Why is it that even in countries with low HIV/AIDS rates, some regions are severely affected while others are not?

These are some of the questions this book seeks to answer. Our goal is to understand who is getting what diseases, where, and why. We will examine the geographic distribution of known diseases, such as tuberculosis (TB), malaria, and HIV/AIDS, as well as recently emerged diseases, such as Ebola, pandemic influenza, and swine flu. Finally, we will look at the potential impact that global climate change has on disease.

GLOBALIZATION AND DISEASE

Over the past two centuries, the average distance and speed of human travel have increased tremendously. What historically may have been only a small, localized outbreak of a disease can now develop in a matter of days into a large, global pandemic. Today, unprecedented numbers of people are also on the move. Three decades ago, there were about 200 million international tourists annually. By 2010, the number increased to 900 million. Airlines carry more than 2 billion passengers each year. Our highly mobile world provides numerous opportunities for the rapid spread of infectious diseases. Thus, a disease outbreak in any one part of the world can spread rapidly to become a threat somewhere else within hours.

Infectious diseases are not only spreading faster, but they appear to be emerging more quickly than ever before. According to the World Health Organization (WHO), newly emerging diseases have been identified at the unprecedented rate of one or more per year since the 1970s. There are now nearly 40 diseases that were unknown a generation ago. New diseases that have been identified recently include HIV, Ebola, Marburg fever, and severe acute respiratory syndrome (SARS). The WHO has confirmed more than 1,100 epidemic events around the world since 2001.

While new diseases keep emerging, diseases previously considered to be controlled have returned, usually with new, more deadly strains. Cholera has come back and is killing hundreds of people in Zimbabwe. Other old threats, such as pandemic influenza, malaria, and tuberculosis, have become more deadly through mutation and growing resistance to antibiotics. SARS and avian influenza have caused major human suffering and economic damage.

Moreover, gains in many areas of infectious disease control have been erased by the spread of drug resistance. For example, extensively drug-resistant tuberculosis (XDR TB) is now a huge problem. Drug resistance is common in diarrheal diseases, malaria, meningitis, and sexually transmitted infections; similar resistance is emerging in HIV.

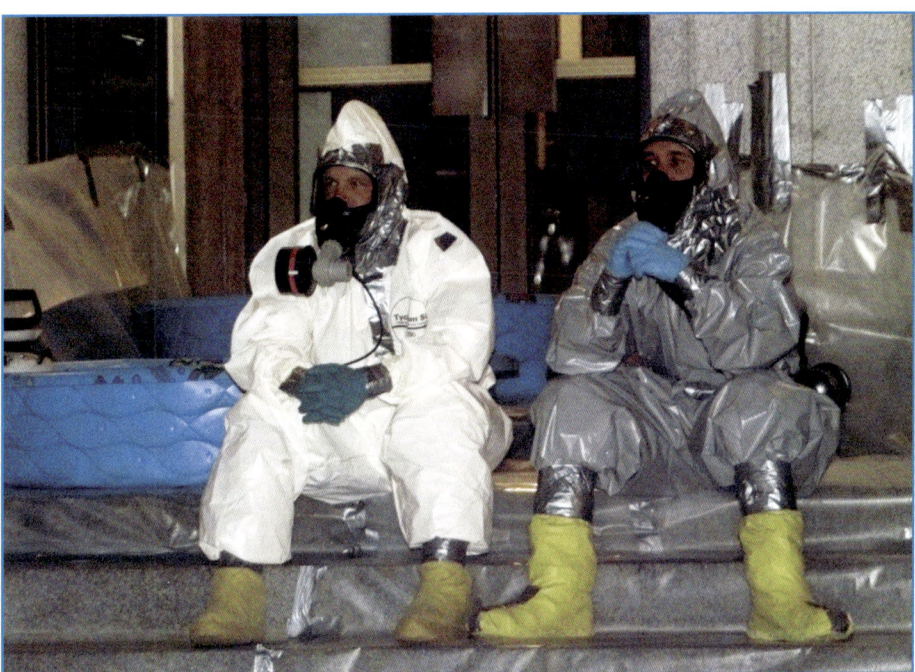

Laboratory technicians wait to be decontaminated after performing an anthrax sweep of the Russell Senate Office Building on Capitol Hill in 2001. The sweep was ordered when Senator Patrick Leahy's office received a suspicious letter. Bioterrorism is a grave threat to global health.

Linked global food production and distribution have made food-borne disease outbreaks from contamination a problem everywhere. In addition, the emergence of new food-borne diseases, such as mad cow disease (bovine spongiform encephalopathy, or BSE), is a major concern.

Bioterrorism, the intentional and cruel release of dangerous pathogens, once unthinkable, has become a reality. Do you remember the anthrax-laced letters distributed in the United States in 2001? Coming only days after the terrorist events of September 11, the deliberate distribution of potentially deadly anthrax spores in letters sent through the U.S. Postal Service was a big shock to many people. Although only 5 people died out of a total of 22 people affected, the anthrax attack had huge economic, public health, and security consequences. The anthrax letters showed that bioterrorism can cause not just death and disability, but it can also cause enormous social and economic chaos. Since the anthrax attacks, many people are now worried that smallpox—eradicated as a human disease in 1979—could be used in vicious new bioterrorist attacks.

In 2003, SARS created even more problems worldwide. SARS was a terrifying disease. It spread from person to person and was not confined to any particular areas. Its symptoms were similar to those of many other diseases. Hospital staff suffered worst of all: About 10 percent of those infected died. The disease spread easily along the routes of international air travel, placing every city with an international airport at risk.

SARS caused much public anxiety, halted travel to affected areas, and caused billions of dollars in economic loss. It raised fears of pandemics to new heights. While poor countries never felt threatened by bioterrorism, every country was concerned about SARS. In fact, SARS showed that the danger arising from emerging diseases is universal. No country, rich or poor, is effectively protected from the arrival of a new disease or the trouble it can cause.

CHOLERA OUTBREAK IN WAR-ZONE IRAQ

On August 20, 2008, the government of Iraq reported the first cholera cases of the year. By September 28, 2008, a total of 341 laboratory-confirmed cholera cases, with 5 deaths, had been verified in 9 provinces. In addition, a further 31 suspected cases and 7 deaths with symptoms similar to those of cholera were under investigation.

The 2008 outbreak appeared to be less intense than previous years, but health experts feared that further waves were still possible. This is because of Iraq's long-term water and sanitation problems. Until access to safe water and proper sanitation is available for all people, cholera outbreaks will recur in Iraq. But how do you ensure safe water and sanitation for everybody in a war zone—a country that is torn by war and violence? Will the roadside bombs and shooting stop so that toilets can be built and water lines can be repaired or installed?

In response to a request from the Iraqi Ministry of Health, the WHO sent a team of health experts to Baghdad, but an assessment mission to Babil and Misan, the most severely affected provinces, had to wait until the security situation improved.

Meanwhile, cholera continued to spread through the country. The world could not stop it. An even bigger concern was that Iraqi refugees would carry cholera to neighboring countries. Iraq's neighbors were encouraged to watch carefully for cholera outbreaks and be prepared to treat their people in case of local outbreaks.

War and violence spread communicable diseases. Not only does war wound and kill people, but it overburdens the health system and destroys the economy. Food supplies are disrupted. Health facilities are sometimes targeted and destroyed to prevent the enemy from using them. Disease prevention efforts such as vaccination programs are disrupted. Land mines used in war maim and kill people, including innocent children. Fleeing war, refugees crowd together amid unsanitary conditions that are ideal for the spread of disease. Can a world that is continually at war avoid global pandemics?

PANDEMICS IN HISTORY: WHY NOW?

When people lived as hunters and gatherers, they were constantly on the move. Disease-causing organisms had trouble keeping up with their human hosts. Once people started living together in larger numbers in the same place, they were more often in contact with their own feces and other wastes for extended periods of time. Poor sanitation, including improper disposal of feces, compounded the problem. Diseases multiplied.

Millions of Roman citizens were killed between A.D. 165 and 180 when smallpox finally reached Rome during the Plague of Antoninus. The bubonic plague hit Europe three centuries later (A.D. 542–543). The Black Death occurred in the fourteenth century when a new route for overland trade with China provided rapid transit for flea-infested furs from plague-ridden China. The Black Death killed up to two-thirds of the population in Europe. In 1855, cholera killed an estimated 500 people in a 10-day period in London. For years, smallpox ravaged populations until it was finally eradicated in 1979. But the best-known global pandemic is the 1918 influenza. It killed between 50 million to 100 million people and sickened one-third of the world's population. In the United States alone, it sickened more than 25 percent of the population and killed more than 600,000 people. This caused the average life expectancy in the United States to drop by 12 years in just one year!

No country in the world has emerged unscathed. Peru has a long and rich history of experience with infectious diseases. Peruvian mummies provide evidence that a TB epidemic occurred 2,000 years ago. Also, Spaniards introduced smallpox into Peru when they first visited the Americas. Peru, in turn, sent syphilis back to sixteenth-century Europe, where Spanish troops spread the epidemic throughout the continent. And it continues today.

Before the 1950s, the disease situation in the world was relatively simple. Only six diseases were a concern: cholera, plague, relapsing fever, smallpox, typhus, and yellow fever. New diseases were rare, and miracle drugs (antibiotics) provided easy cures for many well-known infections. People traveled internationally by ship, and news traveled by telegram. Thus, it took a very long time for diseases to spread around the world.

Since then, the way we live has changed profoundly. Due to rapid population growth, people are living in previously uninhabited areas. Rapid urbanization and increased crowding allow the easy spread of disease. To feed huge populations, farming practices have changed drastically. Intensive farming practices and concentrated animal feeding operations are widespread. The free use of antibiotics and pesticides for both animals and humans has made antibiotic resistance a huge problem. As a result, we now face many new breeds of rapidly spreading super-bugs against which we have little protection.

These threats have become a much larger danger in a world of easy travel. Thanks to the Internet, panic spreads easily with real-time news. Bad health news quickly affects economies and businesses in areas far away from the affected site. Scared, people avoid travel to affected areas. Such reduced travel affects the airlines and tourism, hence, the economies of affected areas. SARS, for example, cost Asian countries about US$60 billion in losses. Sadly, many countries try to conceal disease outbreaks in order to protect their economies. As a result, a disease can spread even more quickly. Ordinary people, unaware of their risk, continue their daily lives without taking appropriate precautions.

Other important factors include reduced public health expenditures, poverty, numerous human conflicts, and poor governments that contribute to each of the foregoing. For a long time, because there were no new infectious disease outbreaks, little was invested in public health. In fact, in the developed countries, some people thought that infectious diseases had been defeated. There was no need to invest in public health then. How wrong they were!

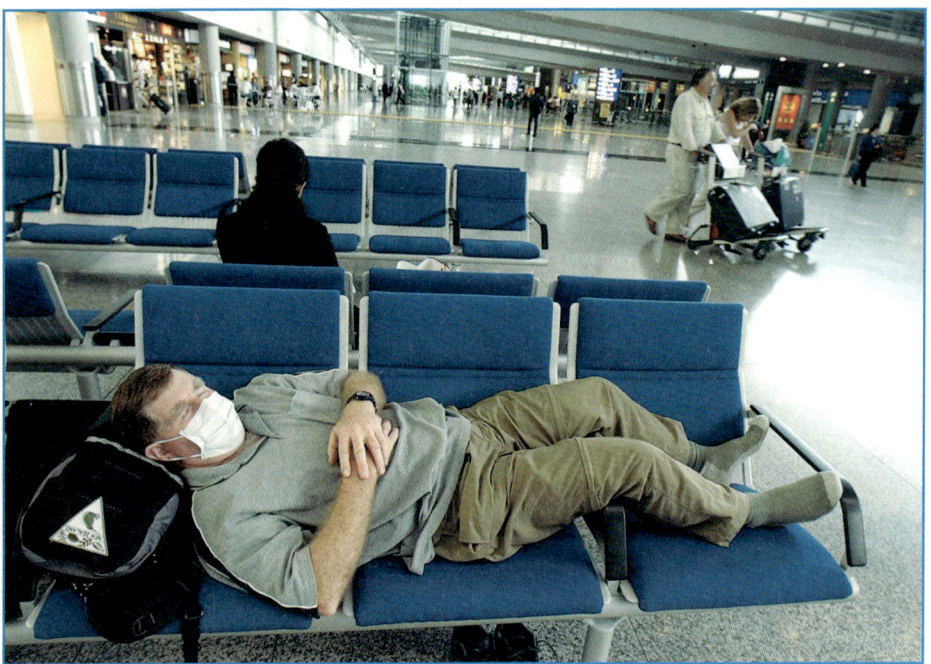

An airline passenger naps in an unusually empty Hong Kong airport in 2003. He wears a mask to protect himself from the SARS virus. The SARS epidemic cost affected countries billions of dollars in lost tourist and business travel.

Numerous wars and other conflicts across the world compound all these problems. Refugees fleeing wars live in poor, overcrowded, and unhygienic communities that increase the risk of epidemics. War makes it difficult to know exactly what diseases are affecting people. In fact, war disrupts needed public health programs, such as immunizations. Diseases like polio continue to spread in conflict-ridden areas of the world such as Pakistan. Throughout most parts of the world, however, it has been almost eradicated. Conflict areas act like reservoirs, making it difficult to overcome and eliminate such diseases.

Finally, poverty has increased throughout the world, especially in developing countries. Poor people have little access to food, clean water, and health care; they live in crowded and unsanitary places that encourage disease spread. With poor nutrition, people are less able to resist infections. Sadly, uncontrolled disease in poor regions of the world puts every living human being at risk. The events of the last two decades show clearly that no country can fully protect its citizens in isolation or through traditional border controls. Clearly, the world needs better health systems. It also needs increased global cooperation and greater vigilance to manage the risks and consequences of the international spread of new infectious diseases.

GLOBAL COLLABORATION IS CRITICAL

The most serious health threats in history usually emerged without warning. Because of this we should expect that another disease like AIDS, Ebola, or SARS will emerge sooner or later. We need effective methods for gathering epidemic disease information and verifying new outbreaks. Rapid field response, including rapid distribution of vaccines and drugs, is desperately needed.

Today, the public health security of people worldwide depends on the ability of each country to act quickly and contribute to the well-being of all. The world is rapidly changing, and today nothing moves faster than information. Sharing essential health information is crucial. Governments can no longer keep outbreaks secret for fear that their economies will suffer disruptions in trade, travel, and tourism.

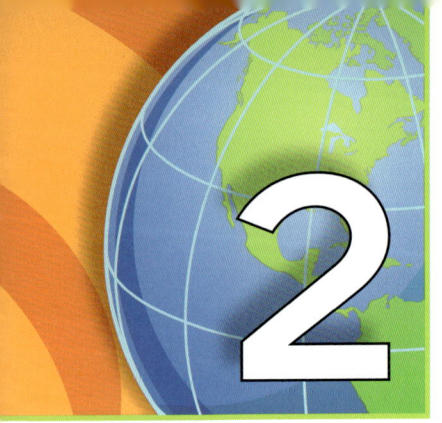

HEALTH GEOGRAPHY AND GLOBAL HEALTH

Getting sick is never fun. If you live in the United States or Canada, or in most European countries, you can easily get medicines that can help you to feel better quickly. For millions of people in developing African and Asian countries, however, getting a disease often means death. This is because the right medicines or treatment facilities are often not available. Diseases such as tuberculosis and even diarrhea, which are easy to cure, still kill many people. Depending on where you live in this world, a simple illness, perhaps caused by an insect bite, can mean life or death. In sickness or health, it matters where you live!

A girl born today can expect to live for more than 80 years if she is born in Sweden or Japan but less than 45 years if she is born in Lesotho or Zimbabwe. The circumstances in which people live and work and the health systems available there are the major reasons for this difference. Political, social, and economic forces, in turn, shape the conditions in which people live and die.

The difference in life expectancy is not just between countries. It is very clear even within countries. In all countries, rich people are usually healthier than the poor because they can afford health care. Poor people have high levels of illness and die much younger than rich people. In fact, poor people usually have worse health in general, but poor people in developing countries have the worst conditions. They lack adequate health care because their governments have so little money to spend on it.

In Canada, poor people actually have good health care because Canada provides health care for all citizens regardless of ability to pay. But in the United States, despite the abundance of excellent health care facilities, poor people who don't have insurance have a tough time getting needed health care. This is because in the United States, health care depends on the ability to pay. Those without insurance have to wait long hours in emergency rooms before they can get care. The rich don't have to wait. They get care easily and quickly in the office of their private doctors. Thus, the health care you get depends on where you live and whether you are rich or poor.

Have you seen images of starving African children on the news? You probably wondered why they were so sickly. In some parts of the world, many children die before their first birthday. In Afghanistan and Sierra Leone, more than 150 out of every 1,000 children born die before their first birthday. In fact, in Angola in 2008, 182 of every 1,000 children born were expected to die within the first year of life. They die of conditions that are easily treated in other parts of the world with excellent health care. In Singapore, Sweden, and Japan, fewer than 3 out of every 1,000 children born were expected to die before their first birthday in 2008. Clearly, where you live in this world makes a big difference in how long you live.

Some parts of the world have abundant food, but other parts do not. Some places are extremely hot; others are extremely cold. Some countries have abundant rainfall; others are parched deserts. Some parts of the world have snow most of the year; others

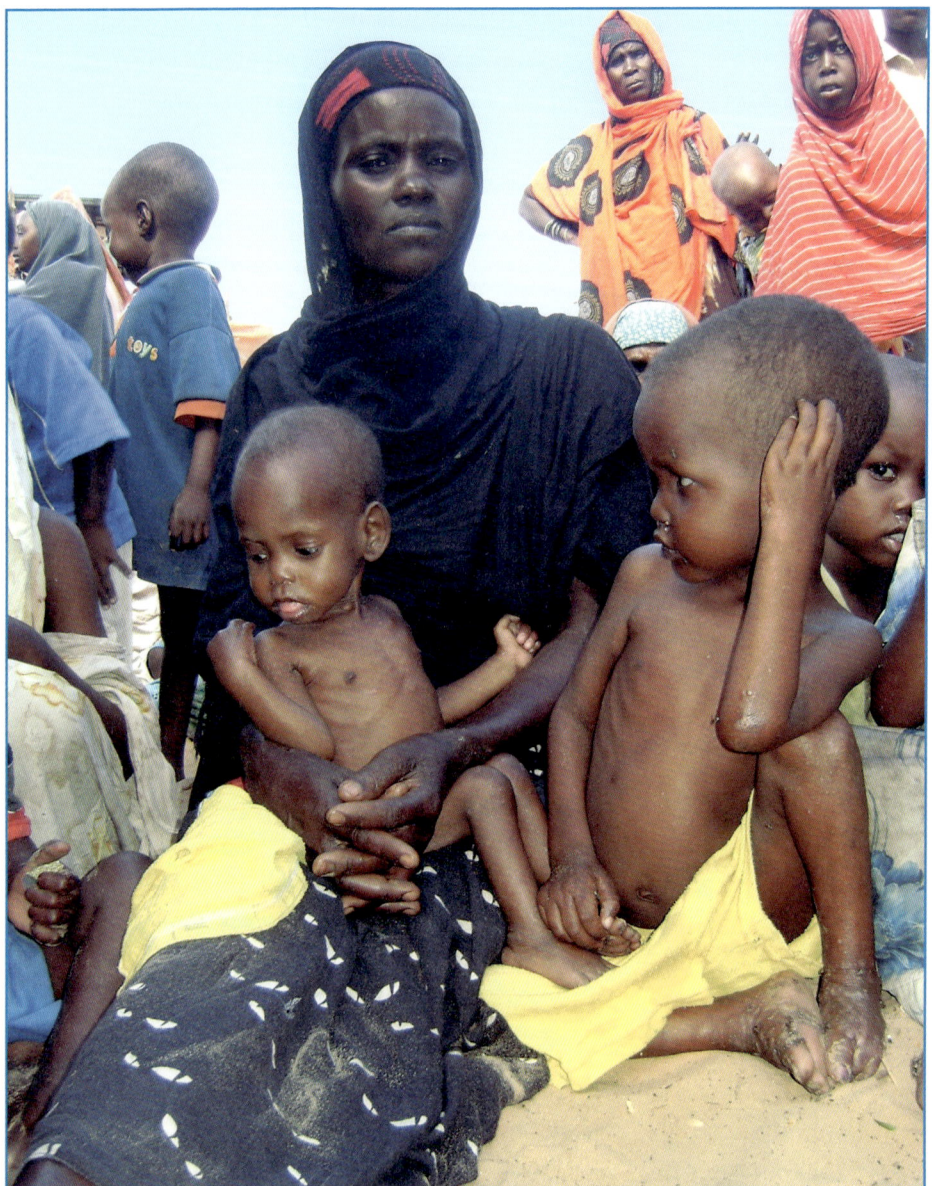

Geography and economics have a critical impact on health care. While some governments provide excellent health care for their citizens, other countries cannot afford to take care of their residents. As a consequence, many children die from conditions and diseases that are easily treated around much of the world.

never see snow. The world we live in varies from one place to another. No two places are exactly the same. People eat different things, experience life differently, and have different cultural values and traditions. All these contribute to differences in health and illness.

Have you ever wondered why some parts of the world seem to have more diseases than others? Why is it that the diseases you hear about in Asia and Africa, such as malaria, are never mentioned in the United States or Canada? Why are some diseases common in one part of the world but completely absent in others? Why do some places have poor health facilities and doctors and other places have excellent health facilities with well-trained doctors?

These are all important questions of health geography and some of the questions we address in this book. We will learn about how and why diseases are spread and health care is distributed around the world. We will explore how the physical environment, including the climate or soil, makes people ill in some places. We will also try to understand how human behavior, such as smoking, makes people sick and how good nutrition and regular exercise make people healthy. Are you ready for a quick tour around the world as we discover what diseases occur where and why? Welcome to the fascinating world of health geography.

HEALTH GEOGRAPHY

Health geographers study why and how diseases and health care vary from one place to another. Using ideas about climate, soil, vegetation, and livelihood, they try to explain who gets what diseases where and why. They also explore the distribution of health facilities and how health care is provided. Health geographers use ideas and concepts from geography in order to understand how health and disease vary from one area to another. Let us begin by explaining some basic terms.

A very important concept in geography is *scale*. In making maps, we represent distances on the ground with smaller distances on a map. For example, one inch on a map may be used to represent one mile on the ground. You will need 100 inches on the map to show two places that are 100 miles apart in real

BAD GOVERNANCE AND CHOLERA IN ZIMBABWE

Zimbabwe provides a classic example of an often neglected cause of communicable disease spread—bad governance. Since August 2008, cholera has ravaged the country. It has killed more than 4,300 people and sickened more than 100,000, with no end in sight.

The country's cholera outbreak is Africa's worst in more than 15 years. Before Zimbabwe's nightmare, Africa's worst experience with the disease was during the mid-1990s. At that time, it killed 12,000 people in camps in what was then Zaire, as refugees fled turmoil following the genocide in Rwanda. What makes Zimbabwe's outbreak unique is that it spread so quickly and has been so deadly in a country at peace.

The cholera was fueled by the collapse of Zimbabwe's water, sanitation, and health systems. Many hospitals had shut down, and many towns had a poor and erratic water supply, broken sewers, and uncollected waste. The political and economic problems facing Zimbabwe have worsened the problem. Many health workers have refused to work unless they are paid in hard currency because the Zimbabwean dollar is virtually worthless.

Cholera is usually easily treated. The scale of Zimbabwe's outbreak is blamed on the collapse of the country's water and health infrastructure following years of violent political impasse. Donors have been slow to provide funds to rebuild that infrastructure because they do not trust president Robert Mugabe. He has been accused of trampling on democracy and ruining a once-thriving economy. Despite formation of a unity government with long-term rivals in February 2009, life. Such a map can show a lot of detail but will involve a huge amount of paper to cover a large area. However, if one inch is used to represent 100 miles, you will need only one inch on the map to show those two places, but you can show only a few details. Generally, small-scale maps—maps where short distances

Mugabe has been slow to act on his promises of reform. The global financial crisis has also slowed foreign aid.

Sadly, President Mugabe denies that there is a cholera problem in Zimbabwe. Despite warnings from the WHO and other organizations, Mugabe has denied the presence of cholera. In a 2008 speech, he said, "They want military intervention, because of cholera. But I'm happy to say that our doctors . . . have now arrested cholera." He is too proud to admit his failures. Meanwhile the people continue to suffer and even die.

Clearly, bad governance spreads disease. It creates economic problems that worsen disease. It also neglects the health care system and other necessary infrastructure like sanitation and health. The problem is that disease in such countries easily spreads to neighboring countries and the world at large. Even worse, such governments conceal the disease outbreak. They deliberately underreport cases to conceal the mess they have created. In such cases, international efforts to control the disease are usually too little too late. From one country disease easily spreads worldwide. Bad governance in one country puts the whole world at risk.

So what should be done to countries that practice bad governance? Should cruel dictators like Mugabe be forcibly removed from power? Whose responsibility is that? What about countries that simply defy the rest of the global community regarding disease risk? Who decides what good governance is and what is not? There are no simple solutions to global disease problems.

on the map represent huge distances on the Earth—show large areas but with very little detail. In contrast, large-scale maps cover small areas of Earth's surface but with lots of detail. In our example, which is the large scale and which is the small scale? When we represent 100 miles with only one inch on the map, we can cover a much larger area but with very little detail. This is a small-scale map. But when one inch represents one mile, we can show a much larger area; this is a relatively large-scale map.

We can also think about scale in terms of the area covered: global scale (around the world), national scale (around the country), or local scale (around you). The global scale covers all countries or areas on the globe—the whole world. At the national scale, we are thinking about our particular country, such as the

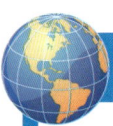

MAKING C◉NNECTI◉NS

THE GLOBAL FOOD WEB

As we sit at the dinner table, pick up a fork, and take a juicy bite of dinner, we hardly think about the huge global connections of the food on our plate. Our beef comes from Iowa, fed by Nebraska corn. Our grapes come from Chile, our bananas from Honduras, our olive oil from Sicily, and our apple juice not from Washington state but all the way from China. Your chocolate bar snack includes cocoa from Ghana or Ivory Coast, and your dad's coffee is from Kenya or Colombia. Did you know that Starbucks carries Rwandan coffee?

Modern society has relieved us of the burden of growing, harvesting, even preparing our daily food, in exchange for the burden of simply paying for it. Only when prices rise do we take notice. And the consequences of our inattention are profound. The global food web eases global disease spread. Is your food safe? How can we prevent global food contamination?

United States, Canada, or Mexico. Finally we can think about the local scale, maybe our county, zip code, town, or city. While these distinctions are very useful, it is important to remember that they are not marked on the ground; they are just concepts or ideas for our discussion. Some diseases are local diseases; others are global. HIV/AIDS is a global disease, but some disease outbreaks may be just local. Let us look at a recent local outbreak of disease.

In 2008, about 180 people who ate at a Mexican restaurant near Kent State University in Kent, Ohio, became sick afterward. Health officials began investigating the outbreak after people started arriving at local emergency rooms complaining of diarrhea and severe vomiting. Many of those affected were Kent State students who had eaten burritos at the restaurant. Some had been given coupons for free food at the restaurant for donating blood. Health officials investigating the outbreak said it could be from food-borne bacteria—like salmonella—or a virus spread by a sick restaurant worker. To stop it, the restaurant reopened with employees from other store locations, replaced its food supply, and sanitized all equipment.

Sometimes, a local outbreak can become a national outbreak if, for example, the source of the outbreak distributes contaminated food nationwide. A 2009 local salmonella outbreak in Washington state became a national outbreak before it was contained. Salmonella bacteria live in the intestines of people and animals. Food outbreaks typically are caused by direct contamination of foods that are eaten raw or not fully cooked. Fever, diarrhea, and abdominal cramps typically start 8 to 48 hours after infection and can last a week. Many people recover without treatment. But severe infection and death are possible. About 95 people were hospitalized in the salmonella outbreak, which caused illnesses in 36 states, including Washington, D.C. The U.S. Food and Drug Administration blamed the outbreak on contaminated tomatoes that were distributed nationwide.

Finally, some diseases are global in scope. They affect people in almost every country. HIV/AIDS, influenza, and tuberculosis are excellent examples. In fact, due to increased ease, frequency, and speed of worldwide travel, local disease outbreaks easily become global outbreaks.

Let's look at a simple example of how global travel spreads disease. A man who lives in Texas visits his friends in Ghana. The air portion of his trip begins at Dallas-Fort Worth International Airport. From there he flies to Heathrow International Airport in London, England, before traveling from London to Accra, Ghana. His flight to London takes nine hours, and he has to wait another four hours in London before the Accra flight, which takes another six hours. Suppose the man had some infectious disease that spreads easily through the air as he exhales. Can you imagine the number of people that would be exposed? Obviously, most of the people on the Dallas–London flight would be exposed as well as the people on the London–Accra flight. The same thing would be repeated on the man's return flight. In addition, most people in the transit terminal who sat near him would be exposed to the infection. Thus, the infection can easily and quickly spread to the ends of the world. This happens more frequently than we think.

National Salmonella Outbreak in the United States

In January 2009, U.S. health officials investigated a salmonella outbreak that had sickened nearly 500 people in 43 states, with more than 100 hospitalizations. Ohio officials reported that at least 50 people had been sickened. California officials reported 51 cases, and another 20 were reported in Michigan. Salmonella outbreaks through tomatoes, peanut butter, and even chilies are well known. This latest outbreak was traced to peanut butter and peanut paste made at a peanut processing plant in Blakely, Georgia.

Most people infected with salmonella develop diarrhea, fever, and abdominal cramps 12 to 72 hours later. The illness usually lasts four to seven days. Most people recover without treatment.

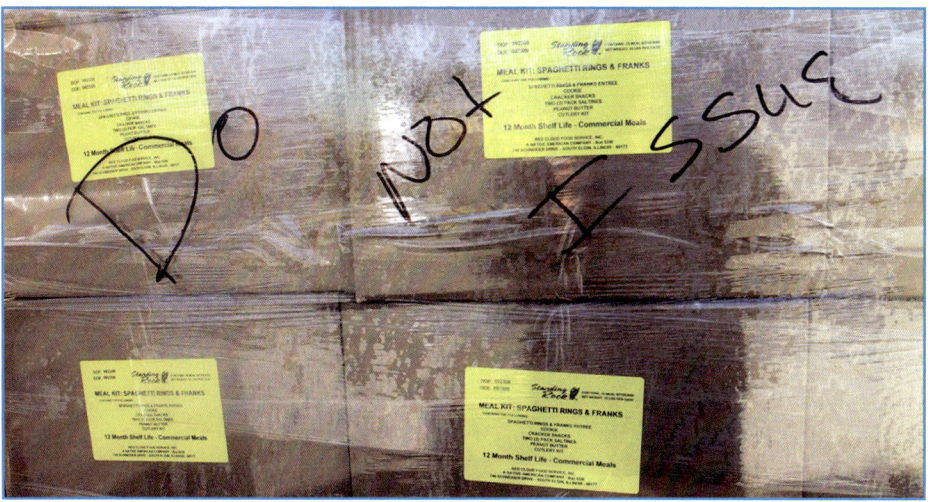

A skid of meals ready to eat (also known as MREs) set to be distributed by FEMA to victims of an ice storm is marked "Do Not Issue" due to concerns that the kits contained contaminated peanut butter. While many people became sick from the 2009 salmonella outbreak, the situation would have been much worse if officials had not discovered and contained the tainted products.

To find out how they got sick, the Centers for Disease Control and Prevention (CDC) interviewed 57 people ill with the outbreak strain of salmonella and compared their food-consumption histories to 399 healthy people. They learned that sick people tended to have eaten brands of peanut butter crackers already linked to contaminated peanut paste. Adults and children sickened at hospitals, nursing homes, and schools tended to have eaten the same brand of peanut butter. In all 14 institutions for which detailed information was available, salmonella illnesses were traced to the single brand of peanut butter.

The most damning evidence came from Connecticut, where on January 19 an unopened jar of the peanut butter was found to contain the same *Salmonella typhimurium* bacteria isolated from sick people. Earlier, the same strain of salmonella was found in an opened jar of the peanut butter in Minnesota. After health investigators isolated salmonella in two places inside the processing plant, it was shut down and most of the products were recalled.

Can you imagine what would have happened if the Georgia plant had shipped some contaminated peanut products overseas? How many people would have gotten sick? How many would have died? Where would they be? In areas with poor health systems, maybe many more people would have died. However, areas that do not receive such peanut butter would not have any salmonella problems.

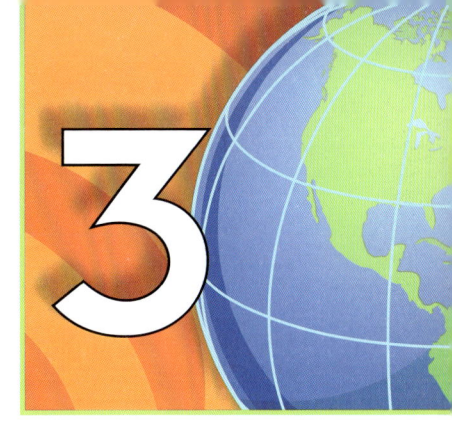

PANDEMICS, EPIDEMICS, AND ENDEMICS

An endemic disease is one always present in an area. For example, large parts of Africa are endemic for malaria. The reason for this is quite simple. Malaria is carried by the female anopheles mosquito, which thrives in warm, moist tropical environments. When the mosquito draws a blood meal from a person with malaria, it spreads the illness to its next victim. Thus, there are only two ways to eliminate malaria. Either all mosquitoes in an area must be killed at once, or all people infected with the disease must be cured so the disease cannot spread.

So far, neither approach has been successful in Africa. Pesticide-resistant mosquitoes have emerged and are thriving. Drug-resistant strains of malaria also appear to be widespread in African countries. And the physical environment (high temperature and standing water) and cultural practices, such as farming, combine to create an environment in which mosquitoes thrive.

An epidemic is a sudden, severe outbreak of disease. It may be local or regional, but the number of infected people is usually much more than expected based on recent experience. An excellent example is diabetes in the United States. Once recognized as a disease that affected only a small number of people, today more than 18 million Americans suffer from this disease. The 2008 cholera outbreak in Zimbabwe is another example. It started in August 2008. By January 30, 2009, more than 60,000 people had been infected and more than 3,000 had died from the disease. Similar outbreaks of cholera and other diseases occur regularly in refugee camps and frequently sicken or kill hundreds of people.

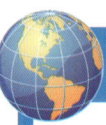

MAKING C⊕NNECTI⊕NS

AMERICA'S OBESITY EPIDEMIC

The United States has a huge problem with childhood and adult obesity. And it is not going away. In 2008, it was reported that adult obesity rates rose in 23 of the 50 states but fell in none. Obesity affects 34 percent of adults aged 20 and older in the United States. In addition, the percentage of obese and overweight children exceeded 30 percent in 30 states. That means one in three children in 30 states is obese! Obese children become obese adults with huge chronic disease problems.

Obesity is linked to a range of health problems, including heart disease, stroke, and type 2 diabetes. That means widespread obesity, as experienced in the United States, fuels high rates of chronic disease prevalence and is responsible for a large and growing chunk of the skyrocketing domestic health care costs. In fact, as obesity increases and waistlines grow, so do health care costs.

Can you think about the implications of the obesity problem for the U.S. economy? In the same way that an obese and unhealthy person can't run as fast as someone who is not obese, the United States may not be able to compete with a global workforce that is healthier and less obese. Unless Americans do something quickly about obesity,

An international outbreak of disease is called a pandemic. HIV/AIDS is the world's best-known pandemic. Every country in the world has been affected. About 33.2 million people were living with HIV in 2007. More than 2.1 million people died of AIDS that year. Overall, more than 25 million people have died of AIDS since 1981.

The term *pandemic* emphasizes geographic spread, not the number of cases or severity of the disease. For example, the World Health Organization (WHO) declared the H1N1 virus (swine flu) pandemic in June 2009. At that time, it had killed

the economy will begin to suffer because it is weighed down by bad health.

Obesity is growing very rapidly in the United States. In 1991, no state had an adult obesity rate above 20 percent, and in 1980, the national average for adult obesity was 15 percent. Can you imagine what the obesity rates will be 10 or 20 years from now if the patterns do not change? Childhood obesity rates in the United States have more than tripled since 1980, and they continue to grow. Parts of the rest of the world seem to be catching up: In Europe, Australia, New Zealand, and the Middle East, the occurrence of obesity appears to be increasing. In 2008, the levels ranged between 10 and 20 percent.

What would happen if all Americans started eating healthy and exercising regularly? Health care costs could come down, but the cost of nutritious food would probably increase significantly. Poor people would be less able to afford such healthy food, and the obesity epidemic would probably increase. Imagine what would happen when these obese children become adults. Even more scary, consider an astronomical increase in obese adults aged 65 and older. Could America handle that? Who will take care of aging, obese, and unhealthy America?

fewer than 200 people, but it had spread to 74 countries. Some people even say that obesity has become a global pandemic. It is a problem all over the world. A 2000 study of Australians showed that more than 60 percent of adults and 20 percent of children were overweight or obese.

Diseases are referred to as chronic when they are present or recur over a long period of time. Diabetes and heart disease are excellent examples of chronic disease. Health-damaging behaviors such as tobacco use, lack of exercise, and poor eating habits are major contributors to the leading chronic diseases. Chronic diseases tend to become more common with old age.

Diseases are called acute when their symptoms are severe and their course is brief. This is the opposite of chronic diseases. Examples of acute diseases include colds. Some acute diseases may not require significant treatment. For example, an individual may recover from influenza at home, without taking prescription medications or requiring the care of a physician.

Disease incidence and disease prevalence do not mean the same thing. Incidence refers to the number of new cases of a disease reported or diagnosed during a set period, usually one year. Prevalence refers to the total number of people in a population sick with that disease at a particular time. Thus, the incidence of tuberculosis refers to the number of new cases diagnosed this year, whereas the prevalence refers to the total number of people living with the disease. It doesn't matter when they were diagnosed.

An infectious disease results when an infectious agent invades the body and its activities cause disease that can be transmitted to other individuals. The agent can be a virus, bacteria, or parasite. For example, measles is infectious because it occurs when an individual contracts the measles virus. The infected person passes it on to others who come in contact with him or her. Infectious diseases are also called communicable diseases.

Microorganisms that cause disease are called pathogens. When a pathogen invades your body and begins growing in it, you have been infected. Disease results when, as a result of the infection, your body does not function the way it should. Our bodies are designed to prevent infection and, should that fail, to prevent disease after infection occurs.

Some pathogens are very contagious and easily transmitted, but they are not very virulent (that is, they are not very likely to cause disease). For example, the polio virus probably infects most people who contract it, but only about 5 to 10 percent of them actually develop the disease. In contrast, Ebola is very virulent but probably not very contagious. About 50 to 90 percent of those infected with Ebola die. Pathogens that are both very contagious and very virulent are the biggest threat.

DISEASE RESERVOIRS

The reservoir for a disease is the site where the infectious agent survives. For example, humans are the reservoir for the measles virus because it does not infect other organisms. Animals often serve as reservoirs for diseases that infect humans. Swine flu is a good example. Also, wildlife is a major reservoir for many diseases that affect humans and domestic animals. People working with wildlife should be alert to the potential for disease transmission from animals. There are also nonliving reservoirs. Soil is the reservoir for many disease-causing fungi and bacteria, such as the bacteria that cause tetanus.

Sometimes, the reservoir of a disease may be unknown. A good example is Buruli ulcer. Although it is caused by a mycobacterium similar to what causes tuberculosis (TB), scientists have yet to identify its reservoir. We know that people who live close to water bodies in low-lying elevations with swampy vegetation in tropical regions have higher rates of the disease. But scientists have no clue how it was transmitted to humans. Is it through an insect bite? Is it through soil exposure? Or through entry into an open wound or sore? Nobody knows yet. Even more mysterious is the fact that all members of a family that eat the same food, farm, and live together may not be affected. In one family sometimes only one person is affected. Scientists are still working to find an answer.

There is concern that many disease-causing organisms are lurking out there in forests and other areas that have not been altered by humans. As humans move into these areas, they become exposed and may develop these diseases.

HOW DISEASE SPREADS

Pathogens may be transmitted through direct or indirect contact. Direct contact occurs when an individual is infected by contact

BURULI ULCER: AN ENVIRONMENTAL DISEASE?

Buruli ulcer is an example of a newly emerged disease that may be due to human modification of the physical environment. It is caused by a mycobacterium similar to what causes TB and leprosy, and it has become an important cause of human suffering in Africa since 1980. Buruli ulcer destroys the skin and underlying tissues and produces large skin ulcers that cause deformities. Most patients are women and children who live in rural areas near rivers or wetlands. The exact mode of transmission remains unknown.

In Africa, the disease was first detected in Uganda, but it is now present in many countries. In the Ivory Coast, up to one-sixth of the population in some villages is affected. Very high rates have been reported in Benin, Ghana, Cameroon, and the Democratic Republic of Congo. Probably most cases are not reported. Outside Africa, Buruli ulcer cases have been reported in Australia, China, and Brazil.

Buruli ulcer often starts as a painless swelling in the skin. The pathogen produces a toxin, which destroys skin tissue while suppressing the immune system. Because Buruli ulcer is minimally painful, those affected do not seek prompt treatment. Ultimately, massive areas of skin and with a disease reservoir. Examples include touching an infected person, as happens with chicken pox; eating infected meat; or being bitten by an infected animal (for example as in rabies) or insect (as in the case of ticks and Lyme disease). Transmission by direct contact also includes inhaling a pathogen in droplets from a sneeze or cough, such as with tuberculosis. Another example is when a pathogen is spread through intimate sexual contact. Some diseases that are transmitted primarily by direct contact include ringworm, AIDS, influenza, and rabies.

Indirect contact occurs with a pathogen that can survive outside its host for a long period of time before infecting another individual. Contaminated objects like a tissue used to wipe the

sometimes even bone are destroyed. That is why it is sometimes called skin-eating bacteria. The disease causes gross deformities, extensive scarring, restricted movement of limbs, and permanent disabilities.

No cure currently exists. The only viable treatment as of 2007 was surgery followed by a skin graft. This is a costly procedure that is not easily available to those affected by the disease. After all, many of them live in areas with limited access to health services. Also, many patients seek treatment too late.

Environmental modification, including deforestation, dam and road building, and farming and mining, has been associated with a higher prevalence of the disease. For example, in Benin, the rate of Buruli ulcer in environmentally modified areas was 180 per 100,000 compared to 20 per 100,000 in other areas. That is why some researchers blame human activities. They claim that as humans seek more and more land, they extend into areas occupied by previously unknown pathogens. These pathogens then cause new diseases. Some aquatic insects have also been blamed. (For additional information, go to http://www.who.int/gtb-buruli/.)

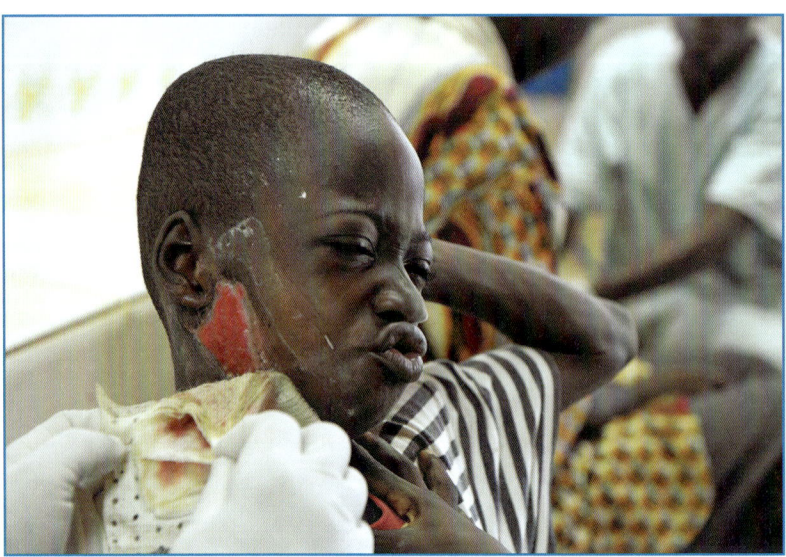

A West African child suffering from Buruli ulcer is treated at a clinic in 2009. Since the first case was diagnosed in 1978, the Ivory Coast has been most affected by the rapidly spreading disease, with approximately 30,000 cases.

nose of a person with a cold may spread the cold virus. Similarly, a toy that has been handled by a sick child may be the indirect contact for disease spread. Eating food and drinking beverages contaminated by contact with a sick person are other examples. Using sewage-contaminated water for drinking, washing, or preparing foods is a major form of indirect transmission. This is why poor sanitation is frequently blamed for many diseases in developing countries. These methods of transmission are all examples of horizontal transmission because the infectious agent is passed from person to person in a group.

Some diseases also are transmitted vertically. That is, they are transmitted from parent to child during the processes of reproduction (through sperm, egg cells, or birth). AIDS is a disease that is transmitted vertically. An infant contracts the disease before birth from his or her mother. Or an infant can get it from his or her mother's breast milk. The herpes virus may also be transmitted to a baby during vaginal birth.

DEGENERATIVE DISEASES

Unlike infectious diseases, degenerative diseases are caused by the aging process. Heart attacks and strokes are more common in older people. They occur later in life after lifestyle decisions have led to cholesterol buildup that limits blood circulation. Degenerative diseases are not infectious. They can't be passed from one person to another. You don't get heart disease from touching a person with heart disease. Similarly, you can't get diabetes from contact with a diabetic. However, if you adopt the lifestyle and behavior of a person with a degenerative disease, including his or her diet habits and lack of exercise, you may be more likely to get a degenerative disease.

THE HISTORY OF MEDICINE

In medieval times, most people believed that supernatural forces created diseases to punish humans for their bad behavior and sins. Around 1530, it was discovered that diseases could be contagious. That is, they could be transmitted by direct contact with an infected person, contaminated materials, or infected air. Microorganisms were discovered around the late 1600s and were subsequently seen as the cause of disease.

Although the germ theory of disease was first proposed in 1762, it was fully developed by Robert Koch in the 1870s as he studied anthrax, a disease that affects animals and sometimes humans. After this initial work on anthrax, scientists identified the infectious agents involved in many bacterial diseases. Yet, the causes of many other diseases remained elusive.

In 1900, Walter Reed discovered that a virus caused yellow fever in humans. The work of Koch, Reed, and other researchers led to an understanding of the viral basis of many diseases. The development of more sophisticated biochemical techniques in the early 1900s revealed the chemical simplicity of viruses. And the invention of the electron microscope in 1932 allowed viruses to be seen for the first time. Here are some important dates and names in the history of medicine.

DISEASE	YEAR DISCOVERED	SCIENTIST
Anthrax	1876	Robert Koch
Gonorrhea	1879	Albert Neisser
Tuberculosis	1882	Robert Koch
Plague	1894	Kitasato Shibasaburō Alexandre Yersin
Whooping cough	1906	Jules Bordet Octave Gengou

Vaccination began in the 1700s. A rural English physician, Edward Jenner, observed that his patients who had contracted and recovered from cowpox, a disease similar to smallpox, seemed to be immune not only to further cases of cowpox but also to smallpox. By scratching the fluid from cowpox lesions into the skin of healthy individuals, he was able to immunize those people against smallpox. Louis Pasteur later developed vaccines for anthrax and rabies. Vaccination is now used to immunize people against many diseases.

A key step forward in the fight against infectious disease was the discovery and development of drugs that could kill the microbe involved without killing the patient. Antibacterial drugs were discovered first. In 1929, Alexander Fleming discovered penicillin. Later, in the early 1940s, a group of British scientists showed that penicillin was effective in controlling some infectious diseases and developed procedures for its mass production. The pharmaceutical industry flourished after World War II, and many additional antibiotics were discovered or developed.

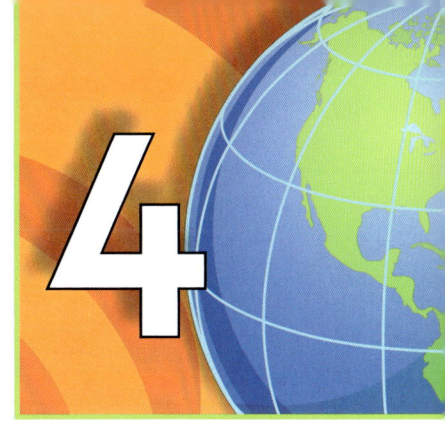

HIV/AIDS

HIV/AIDS is currently the world's most serious communicable disease. It has killed more than 25 million people since it was first discovered in 1981. It continues to spread around the world like wildfire. It leaves behind devastation and misery, including widespread poverty and millions of AIDS orphans. Despite serious efforts and investment in research, there currently is no cure for the disease. In 2007, about 33 million people worldwide were living with HIV. It killed 2.1 million people that year, and 2.5 million were newly infected.

Although every country in the world has been affected by HIV/AIDS, none has suffered more severely than the countries of sub-Saharan Africa. By December 2007, 68 percent of the world's people living with HIV/AIDS (about 22 million people) were in sub-Saharan Africa. That is also where 68 percent of new infections and 76 percent of deaths occur. Unlike other world regions where men have higher rates, women and children in sub-Saharan Africa are far more severely afflicted by the disease. Of those

Africans living with HIV, 61 percent are women, and 90 percent of all HIV-positive children in the world are in sub-Saharan Africa.

Within Africa, southern Africa is by far the most afflicted. It has one-third of all new HIV infections globally and one-third of all people living with HIV/AIDS. In eight countries—Botswana, Lesotho, Mozambique, Namibia, South Africa, Swaziland, Zambia, and Zimbabwe—national adult HIV-prevalence rates exceed 15 percent.

HIV is spread through the exchange of bodily fluids, for example, through sexual activity or intravenous drug use. This

REGIONAL STATISTICS FOR HIV/AIDS, END OF 2007				
Region	Adults and Children Living With HIV/AIDS	Adults and Children Newly Infected	Adult Prevalence	Deaths of Adults and Children
Sub-Saharan Africa	22.0 million	1.9 million	5.0%	1.5 million
North Africa and Middle East	380,000	40,000	0.3%	27,000
Asia	5 million	380,000	0.3%	380,000
Oceania	74,000	13,000	0.4%	1,000
Latin America	1.7 million	140,000	0.5%	63,000
Caribbean	230,000	20,000	1.1%	14,000
Eastern Europe and Central Asia	1.5 million	110,000	0.8%	58,000
North America, Western and Central Europe	2.0 million	81,000	0.4%	31,000
Global Total	33.0 million	2.7 million	0.8%	2.0 million

means that sex workers and people with multiple sexual partners have much higher rates of infection. All over the world, sexually active teens and youth have a very high risk of getting HIV through unprotected sexual activity. Sadly, many people in this age group do not see themselves at risk.

WHAT ARE HIV AND AIDS?

HIV stands for human immunodeficiency virus. This is the virus that causes AIDS, or acquired immunodeficiency syndrome. The virus attacks the human immune system and leaves the body unable to defend itself against many infections. Many common bacteria, yeast, parasites, and viruses ordinarily do not cause serious disease in people with healthy immune systems. But they can easily kill people with AIDS.

HIV has been found in saliva, tears, blood, semen, vaginal fluid, and breast milk. However, only blood, semen, vaginal secretions, and breast milk generally transmit the infection to others. Thus, the virus can be transmitted:

- Through any type of sexual contact
- Through blood, via blood transfusions (now extremely rare in the United States) or needle sharing
- From mother to child. A pregnant woman can transmit the virus to her unborn baby through their shared blood circulation, or a nursing mother can transmit it to her baby in her milk during breast-feeding. This is an excellent example of vertical transmission.

Other transmission methods are rare and include accidental needle injury, artificial insemination with infected donated semen, and organ transplantation with infected organs.

HIV infection is not spread by casual contact such as hugging, by touching items previously touched by a person infected with the virus, during participation in sports, or by mosquitoes.

It is not transmitted to a person who donates blood or organs. However, HIV can be transmitted to a person receiving blood or organs from an infected donor. To reduce this risk, blood banks and organ donor programs screen donors, blood, and tissues thoroughly. In all these procedures, sterile needles and instruments are used in the United States and other developed countries. In developing countries, however, the story may be quite different.

People at highest risk for getting HIV include:

- Intravenous drug users who share needles
- Infants born to mothers with HIV who don't receive HIV therapy during pregnancy
- People engaging in unprotected sex
- People who received blood transfusions or clotting products between 1977 and 1985 (before standard screening for the virus began)
- Sexual partners of those who participate in high-risk activities

AIDS begins with HIV infection. People infected with HIV may have no symptoms for 10 years or longer. But they can still transmit the infection to others during this symptom-free period. Meanwhile, if the infection is not detected and treated, the immune system gradually weakens, and AIDS develops. Without treatment, almost all people infected with HIV will develop AIDS.

AIDS SYMPTOMS

The symptoms of AIDS are usually infections that do not normally develop in individuals with healthy immune systems. These are called opportunistic infections. Because HIV attacks the immune system, the body's natural ability to defend itself, people with AIDS have little natural defense against infection. They become like a city without walls; they are easily overrun by the enemy. Common symptoms of AIDS are fevers, sweats (particularly at night), swollen glands, chills, weakness, and weight loss.

Initial infection with HIV can produce no symptoms. Some people, however, do experience flu-like symptoms with fever, rash, sore throat, and swollen lymph nodes usually two weeks after contracting the virus. Some people with HIV infection remain without symptoms for years between exposure to the virus and the onset of AIDS.

A good measure of a healthy immune system is the number of CD4 cells per milliliter of blood. CD4 cells are immune cells. They are also called T cells or helper cells. A person is diagnosed as having AIDS if he or she has a CD4 cell count below 200. AIDS may also be diagnosed if a person develops one of the numerous infections and cancers that occur with HIV infection. The most common of these infections include tuberculosis and herpes.

While there is no cure for AIDS at this time, many available treatments can help to reduce or suppress the symptoms. This allows people to live much longer with a much higher quality of life. Antiretroviral therapy suppress the replication of the HIV virus in the body. A combination of several antiretroviral drugs, called highly active antiretroviral therapy (HAART), has been effective in reducing the number of HIV particles in a unit of blood. Preventing the virus from replicating can help the immune system recover from the HIV infection.

Unfortunately, while HAART is widely available in developed countries, few AIDS patients in developing countries have access to these therapies. For example, few Africans living with HIV/AIDS have access to HAART therapies. Yet, Africa is where the bulk of the epidemic is located. In short, those who need HAART the most have the least access to it. This general principle of inequitable access to health resources is called the inverse care law of health. Generally stated, those who need health care the most have the least access to it. Can you think of other examples of the inverse care law in your country or even community?

HAART is not a cure for HIV. People on HAART can still transmit HIV to others through sex or sharing needles during intravenous drug use. Also, HIV may become resistant to HAART in patients who do not take their medicines regularly. When this happens, other drug combinations must be used and control becomes more difficult. Common side effects of HAART treatment include nausea, headache, and general bodily weakness. Also, when used for a long time, these medications increase the risk of heart attack.

WHY IS HIV/AIDS SO SEVERE IN AFRICA?

Several reasons have been suggested for Africa's excessively high HIV/AIDS problem, but the most common underlying thread is poverty. Other important factors include food shortages, labor migration, and war and civil conflicts. Let us look at these a bit more closely.

Poverty drives many men to leave their wives for long periods to find work in distant places such as the gold mines of South Africa. Isolated from their wives, the men often use sex workers to meet their sexual needs. Because they have multiple sexual partners, sex workers usually have high rates of HIV. Once infected, these men infect their wives when they return home. Also, during the long time their husbands are absent, some wives have relations with other men and risk getting the disease. They usually resort to this in order to earn money to provide much-needed household items such as food. Such women are unable to insist on condom use because they desperately need the money.

In the twenty-first century, rape has become a common weapon of war and civil conflicts. Wartime rape, including taking women and girls as sex slaves, is widespread. It is particularly devastating to the victims because of the social stigma rape carries. Also, of course, it carries the risk of HIV/AIDS. In Islamic cultures, if a woman becomes pregnant through rape,

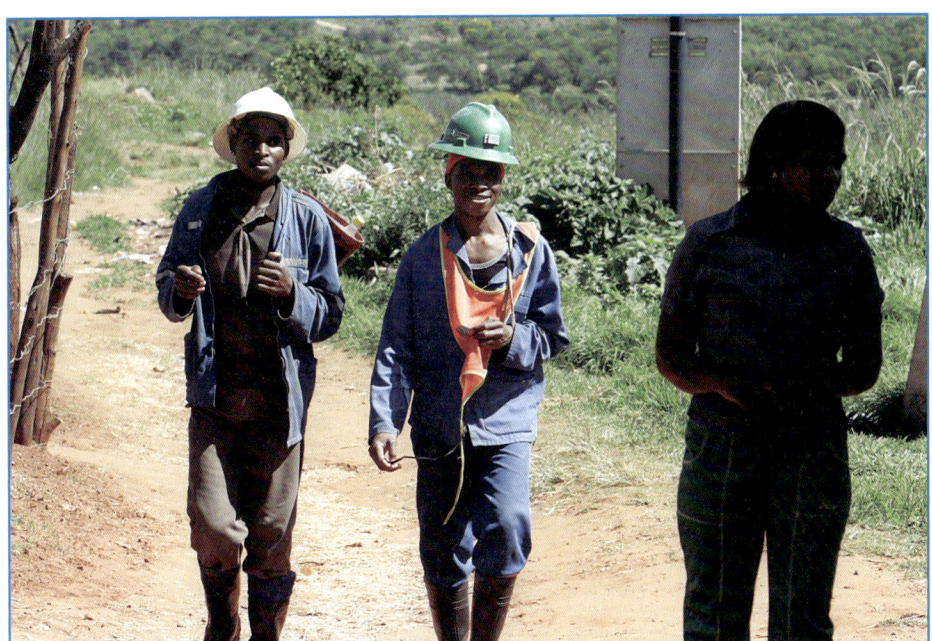

Two miners walk through their squatter settlement in South Africa. Men forced to find work away from their families are at great risk for contracting HIV, due to the lifestyle in such camps.

she may face criminal charges for violating Islamic laws governing extramarital sex. Frequently these women are infected with HIV.

Take the story of Amal, a university student in Darfur. Amal was heading in a van from her hometown to Nyala, Darfur's largest city, where she attends classes at the University of Nyala. On the highway a few hours outside Nyala, about 35 armed men stopped the van. After making the occupants lie on the blistering ground and ransacking the van, the gunmen separated the men from the women. The men were marched off in one direction. The women were taken in another direction, out of sight of passersby, and raped repeatedly at gunpoint for about an hour. Afterward, the victims were let go and their captors disappeared on their camels. Two months later, Amal found that she was pregnant, and she was also diagnosed with HIV. Unfortunately, Amal's story is not unique.

Health care facilities in developing countries are usually poorly equipped and poorly staffed. Due to shortages of supplies and other limitations, blood used for transfusion is not screened thoroughly. Medical equipment, including needles and syringes, is sometimes not adequately sterilized although it is sometimes reused. Moreover, the high cost of HAART means that few African HIV patients obtain these lifesaving drugs. Thus the disease continues to spread its devastation across Africa, with little human resistance.

Until lasting solutions are found for the endemic poverty in African countries, curtailing HIV/AIDS remains only a dream. But eliminating poverty? That is an even bigger problem. Where do you start?

PASCAL'S STORY: LIVING WITH HIV/AIDS IN KENYA

Two-year-old Pascal lives with his mother, Pamela, and father, Charles, in Homa Bay, in western Kenya's Nyanza Province. Pascal is HIV-positive, and so are his mother and father. At seven o'clock every morning, he sits with his mother and father and they all take their morning dose of antiretroviral drugs. They must take a tablet every morning and every evening for the rest of their lives. As soon as he sees the brightly colored tablet in his father's hand, Pascal reaches for it and puts it in his mouth. With a little water he swallows the pill easily. The whole process takes a couple of minutes. Yet it has not always been this way.

Pascal's parents are very fortunate because many people with HIV do not get the lifesaving medications they get. Their expensive medication is provided for free by a nongovernmental organization that provides health care. Pascal has even more to be thankful for. It was only last year that a fixed dose combination (FDC) antiretroviral—one pill that combines the three different drugs needed to treat HIV/AIDS—for children became available. Pascal has been taking them for only a few months. Before that he had to take five different syrups containing the drugs he needs every morning and evening. Getting him to take them was a real struggle. He didn't like the taste of the medicines. Sometimes his parents had to hold him down and force him to take them.

His mother, Pamela, must walk for 40 minutes to obtain medicines at the HIV clinic. She has to carry and store all the different bottles of syrups that Pascal needs. Although the bottles are quite heavy, she prefers to carry the bottles and walk home after her monthly appointments instead of taking public transport. In this part of Kenya, the stigma surrounding HIV is still very strong. Many patients do not want to take public transport carrying the bottles, which will identify that either they or their child is infected with HIV/AIDS. Others cannot afford the 50 cents needed for the journey. For Pamela, with only one child, the walk carrying the bottles is manageable. But for those patients with more than one child, living far from the hospital, it is tough.

Ensuring that the right dosages are given is hard as the different syrups come with different size syringes or measuring cups. Half a syringe from one syrup might be equal to 50 ml, but it could be 25 ml with another. With so many different bottles, and each one requiring a different amount, it is always confusing. "I'm not sure that I always gave him the right amounts," Pamela says.

Giving children the wrong treatment dosage can have serious consequences. But with a limited number of pediatric fixed-dose combinations available in tablet form, most governments use syrups as a way to combine different single-drug formulations. Yet as Pamela's experience shows, the difficulty in taking and giving these syrups can mean that children do not receive the right dosages and do not take their medication properly.

Of the 22 antiretroviral drugs currently available, 8 are not approved for pediatric use and 9 are not available in pediatric formulations. There is a clear and urgent need for more research and development of child-friendly antiretroviral drugs. Such research should focus on creating the best quality drugs possible. It should also emphasize the production of drugs that are easy for children to take.

THE SILENT CRISIS OF AIDS ORPHANS

Africa has a tragic story. The 17 million people who have died from AIDS have left behind 12 million orphans. An AIDS orphan is a child who has lost one or both parents to the disease. What would you do if you lost both of your parents to a dreaded disease? Who would care for you and your siblings? What if there was no family member to take you in and the government couldn't help either because there are too many children like you?

Unfortunately this is the story of 12 million children across Africa. In addition to the trauma of losing their parents, the shame and stigma associated with the disease make life extremely difficult. Most of these children are plunged into desperate poverty when their parents die because no one is available to help them. Some of these AIDS orphans live on the streets and participate in criminal activities in order to survive.

Traditionally, the extended family—aunts, uncles, and grandparents—took care of AIDS orphans. These days, with so many of them, this traditional system is severely strained and there is no place for many of these children in the most severely affected countries. In Zambia, for example, according to USAID statistics, one in every four Zambian children was an AIDS orphan in 2000. Housing, feeding, educating, and nurturing these children is a difficult challenge.

Many children drop out of school with the death of their parents. With no skills because they are so young and can't read or write, their lives become difficult and they are vulnerable. They need food, education, parental guidance, and physical protection. But in Zambia, due to widespread poverty and the severity of the disease, these are difficult to obtain.

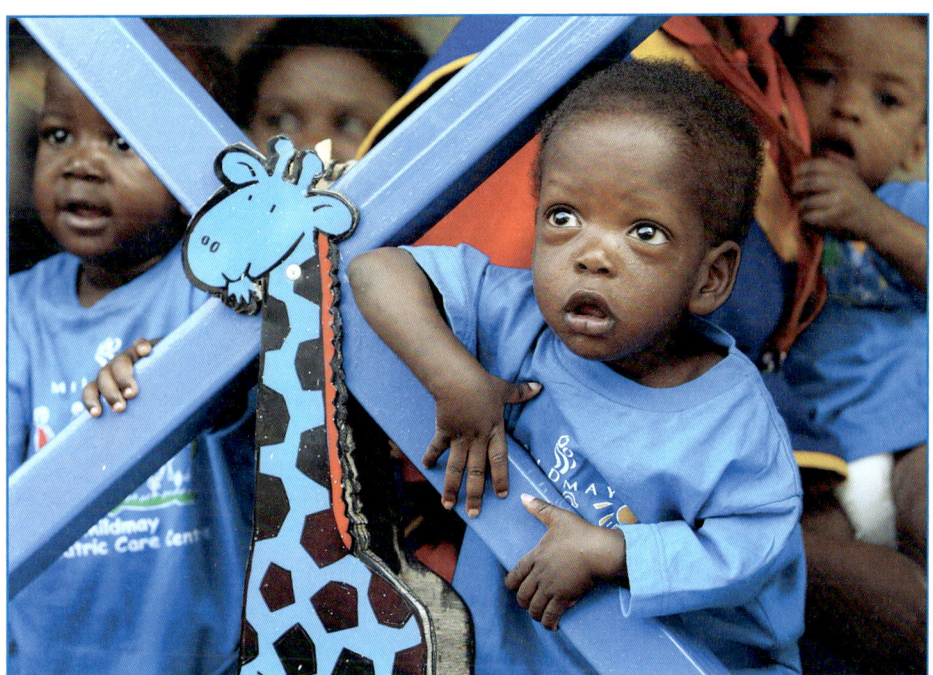

Orphans at the Mildmay HIV Centre in Kampala, Uganda, have been left behind by families that have succumbed to the AIDS epidemic. More than 12 million African children have lost a parent to AIDS.

Part of the problem is financial. The HIV/AIDS pandemic has worsened Zambia's deepening poverty and rising external debt, and it has pushed many families to the very edge of survival. With so many families needing help, this has limited the government's ability to respond to the orphan crisis. Because Zambia has a low per capita income, a mere $800 in 2007, and a huge foreign debt, the government can spend very little on health and education.

For many children, losing their parents brings destitution, an end to schooling, and rejection and shame from their neighbors. The consequences for the family, however, can be devastating. One 70-year-old woman raising her four grandchildren told researchers that "ever since these children were brought to me

I have been suffering. I am too old to look after them properly. I cannot farm anymore because I'm too old and weak. The land is no more fertile land, we can't afford to buy fertilizer, and our meager crop is not enough to feed us."

Child-headed households, once rare in Zambia, are now very common. But inheritance and land ownership laws have not changed to meet their needs. Twelve-year-old Alice is the oldest of five children, the youngest of whom is only two years old. Alice says: "Our parents both died in one year. When this happened, our relatives ran away from us. This surprised us because, being our relatives, we thought they would care for us. . . . Our parents had a big farm, but it was taken from us so we had nowhere to grow food. My young brothers and sisters became beggars; they would walk from house to house asking for food."

Zambia's financial difficulties do not allow the government to provide free education. The government pays teachers' salaries, but local school management committees charge enrollment fees to cover operating costs. In addition, they require school uniforms. Thus, becoming an orphan means an end to education. Without a major increase in financial, technical, and human resources, the future of Africa's orphaned children is bleak.

HIV/AIDS IN THE UNITED STATES

In the United States, HIV/AIDS is not as big a problem as it is in Africa. Less than one percent of the population has AIDS. Even so, most of these people have access to excellent health care and HAART. Thus, most Americans living with AIDS have a very high quality of life and live relatively long lives.

The Centers for Disease Control and Prevention (CDC) estimates that 1.1 million Americans have HIV and that 56,300 new infections occurred in the United States in 2006. However, the HIV epidemic is not uniformly distributed throughout the United

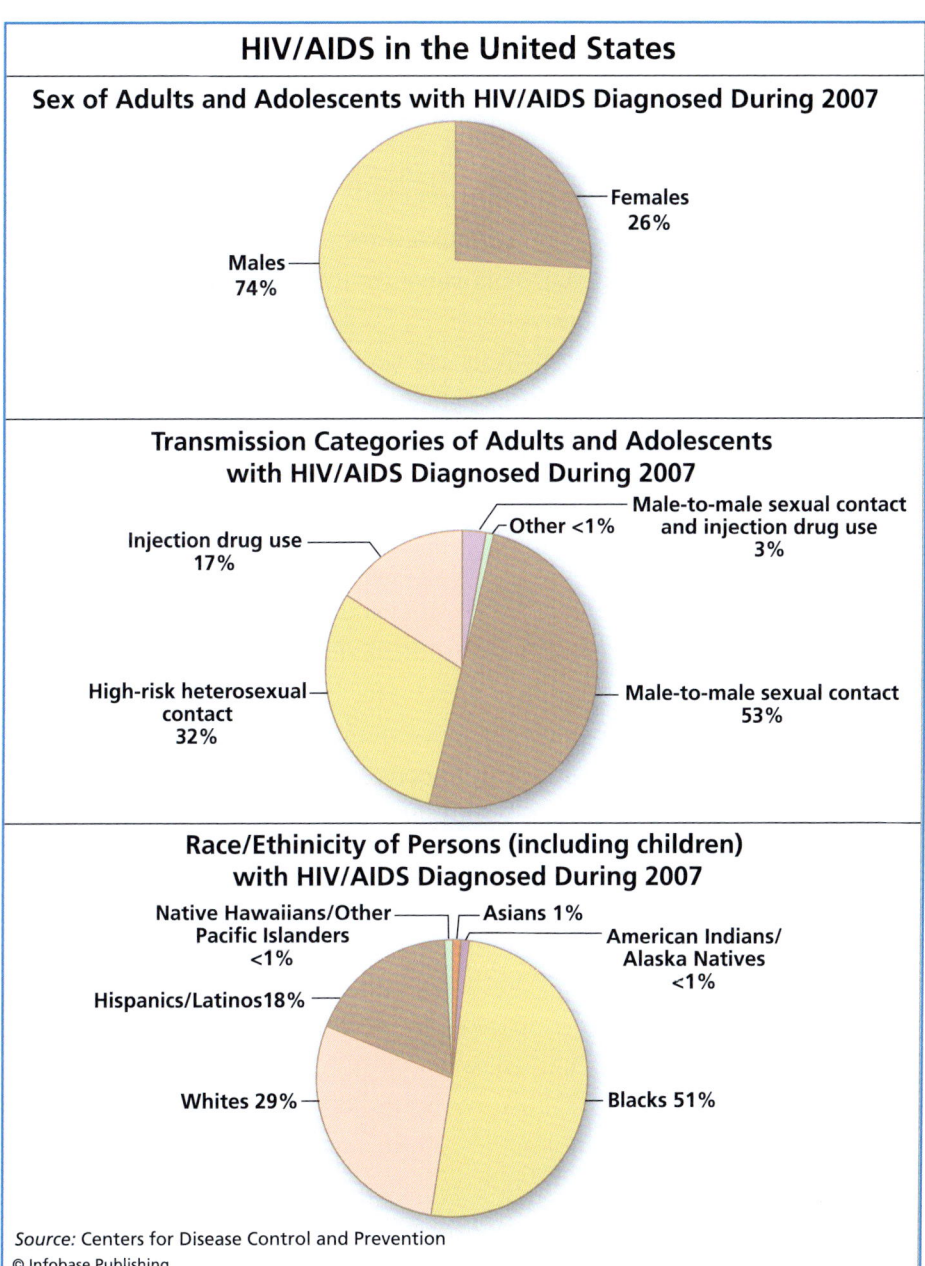

HIV/AIDS in the United States

Sex of Adults and Adolescents with HIV/AIDS Diagnosed During 2007

Females
26%

Males
74%

Transmission Categories of Adults and Adolescents with HIV/AIDS Diagnosed During 2007

Male-to-male sexual contact and injection drug use
3%

Other <1%

Injection drug use
17%

High-risk heterosexual contact
32%

Male-to-male sexual contact
53%

Race/Ethinicity of Persons (including children) with HIV/AIDS Diagnosed During 2007

Native Hawaiians/Other Pacific Islanders
<1%

Asians 1%

American Indians/Alaska Natives
<1%

Hispanics/Latinos18%

Whites 29%

Blacks 51%

Source: Centers for Disease Control and Prevention
© Infobase Publishing

Figure 1.

States (See Figure 1). Nearly 75 percent of HIV/AIDS diagnoses among adolescents and adults in 2006 were for males. The largest proportion of HIV/AIDS diagnoses were for homosexual men, followed by persons infected through high-risk heterosexual contact. African Americans made up only 13 percent of the U.S. population in 2006, yet they accounted for almost half of the estimated number of HIV/AIDS diagnoses made in that year.

Geographic Distribution of HIV/AIDS in the United States

The geography of HIV/AIDS in the United States is quite unusual. Southern states such as Alabama, Mississippi, Louisiana, Florida, South Carolina, and Texas have much higher rates than the rest of the country. Nationally, Georgia ranked fifth in reporting of new AIDS cases in 2007, behind California (first), New York (second), Florida (third), and Texas (fourth). The Northeast also has a heavy burden of HIV/AIDS cases.

U.S. regions with poor access to health care, limited public transportation, and a shortage of doctors have more severe problems. In such areas, people with HIV tend to get tested late, at a time when the disease is advanced. Getting tested soon after infection means treatment can begin early, substantially delaying the development of HIV-related illness and prolonging life. Access to HIV education is also very limited for people in rural areas.

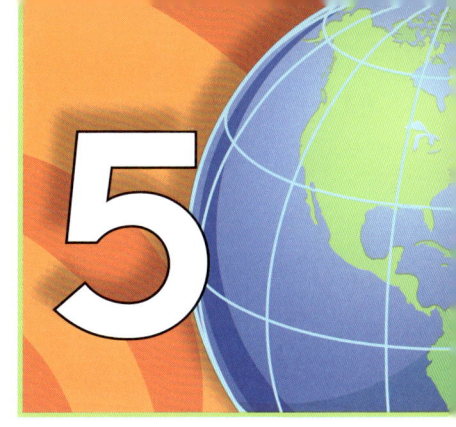

TUBERCULOSIS

Next to HIV/AIDS, tuberculosis (TB) is perhaps the most rapidly spreading infection in the world today, particularly in developing countries. TB bacilli spread when a person with TB coughs, sneezes, speaks, or sings. These pathogens (germs) can float in the air for several hours. When someone inhales the air containing these TB germs, he or she can become infected. Such a person is said to have latent TB.

People with latent TB infection have TB germs in their bodies, but they are not sick because the germs are not active. These people do not have symptoms of TB disease, and they cannot spread the germs to others. This is because their immune systems keep the germs under control. However, they may develop TB disease in the future if the immune system becomes weak from a disease such as HIV/AIDS or even diabetes.

People with TB disease are sick from TB germs that are actively multiplying and destroying tissue in their bodies. They are said to have active TB, and with TB disease of the lungs or throat, they spread it to others. This is why TB is such a huge problem in areas with high HIV/AIDS rates. As we have seen already, HIV weakens your immune system and makes it easy for TB germs to make you sick. The TB germs are much more likely to become active and attack the lungs and other parts of the body.

TB is a curable disease if the infected person takes the prescribed medicine regularly, on time, and completes the dosage. Drug resistance results when the infected person does not complete the medication or misses some doses. Therefore, taking TB medicines exactly as prescribed is the best way to avoid drug resistance.

If infected individuals do not take the drugs correctly, the germs that are still alive may become resistant to those drugs. This means that the medicine can no longer kill the bacteria, making it harder and more expensive to treat.

To help patients remember to take their medications regularly and at the right time, the World Health Organization (WHO) has implemented a special strategy worldwide. Volunteer teams of health workers meet regularly with TB patients to watch them take their medications. This is called directly observed therapy (DOT). DOT helps the patient complete treatment in the least amount of time.

Multidrug-resistant TB, or MDR TB, is caused by bacteria that are resistant to two of the most important TB medicines. A more serious form of MDR TB is called extensively drug-resistant TB (XDR TB). XDR TB is a rare type of TB that is resistant to nearly all medicines used to treat TB disease. People with MDR TB or XDR TB must be treated with special medicines. These medicines are not as effective as the usual medicines for TB and may cause more extreme side effects. Also, treatment takes much longer and people with MDR TB and XDR TB are at greater risk of dying from the disease.

2007 INTERNATIONAL TB SCARE

An Atlanta lawyer caused an international health scare by traveling overseas with what was feared to be extensively drug-resistant tuberculosis. In mid-May 2007, Andrew Speaker flew to Greece to get married and spent his honeymoon in Europe. U.S. health officials found that Speaker had extensively drug-resistant tuberculosis (XDR TB) after he had left for Europe. They tracked him down in Rome and advised him to obtain medical care there.

When he learned of the severity of his illness, he made plans to return to the United States because he was afraid he would die if he did not return to the United States for health care. However, when he found that U.S. health authorities were looking for him, he flew to Canada. From there, he was allowed to cross into New York, even though border guards knew that he should be held for health reasons. Once in New York he voluntarily entered Bellevue Hospital.

Can you imagine how many people were exposed to TB through Speaker? Just think about it for a minute. At the airport, he had to talk to somebody. Going through security he spoke with the transportation security agents. After clearing security, he probably went straight to the boarding gate. Finally, an airline staff member checked him into the flight. He boarded with several other people and was on the flight for hours. All this while, he was breathing, exhaling TB germs into the air. How many people inhaled those? In which countries? At what airports? We probably can never know. Fortunately, after testing, it was confirmed that Speaker did not have XDR TB, the hardest possible variety to cure, as was initially thought. Rather, he had MDR TB, still dangerous but susceptible to more drug treatments.

Speaker's case demonstrates clearly how easily diseases travel between countries and even continents. It shows that diseases do not respect political boundaries. They travel freely and very quickly; they don't need a visa or even a passport. In

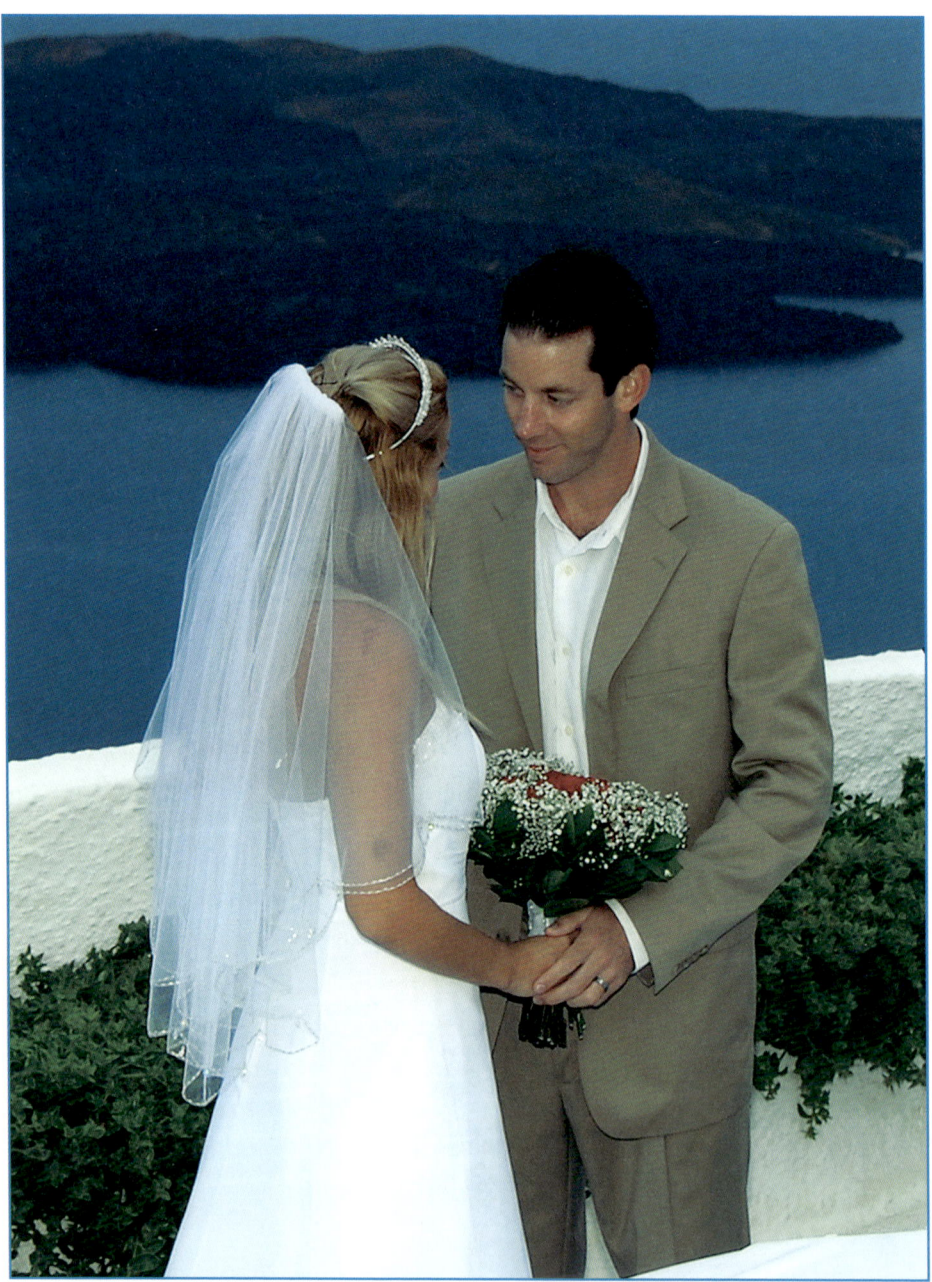

Andrew Speaker marries his bride, Sarah Cooksey, in Greece in 2007. Speaker unwittingly set off a global TB scare when he traveled abroad while infected.

a globalizing world, local disease outbreaks can easily become global outbreaks.

TB is the world's second most significant cause of death due to infection. There were an estimated 13.7 million prevalent cases of TB in 2007 (206 per 100,000 population). Most were in Asia (55 percent) and Africa (31 percent). The five countries that rank first to fifth in terms of total numbers of cases in 2007 were India (2 million), China (1.3 million), Indonesia (0.53 million), Nigeria (0.46 million), and South Africa (0.46 million). Of the 9.27 million cases in 2007, an estimated 1.37 million (14 percent) were HIV-positive; 79 percent of these HIV-positive cases were in Africa and 11 percent were in Southeast Asia.

Although the total number of incident cases of TB is increasing in absolute terms as a result of population growth, the rates are falling slowly. Globally, rates peaked at 142 cases per 100,000 population in 2004. In 2007, there were an estimated 137 incident cases per 100,000 population.

African countries have the highest rates. With only 11 percent of the world's population, Africa has 29 percent of the world's TB cases. The incidence rate in sub-Saharan Africa, estimated by WHO to be 345 per 100,000 population, was double that of Southeast Asia, the next-highest region. Also, in terms of TB incidence, 13 of the world's top 15 countries are in sub-Saharan Africa. Worldwide, an estimated half million cases of multidrug-resistant TB were reported in 2006.

TB IN THE UNITED STATES

In the United States, despite control efforts, all 50 states and the District of Columbia continue to report TB cases. In 2008, a total of 12,898 cases were reported. The TB rate was 4.2 cases per 100,000 in 2007, the lowest rate recorded since national reporting began in 1953. This is much lower than most other parts of the world.

Foreign-born persons and racial/ethnic minorities bear a disproportionate burden of TB disease in the United States. In 2008, the TB rate in foreign-born persons in the United States was 10 times higher than in persons born in the country. This is because most of these people came from developing countries where TB rates are much higher.

TB rates among Hispanics and blacks were nearly 8 times higher than among non-Hispanic whites, and rates among Asians were nearly 23 times higher than among non-Hispanic whites. In 2008, there were 5,283 U.S.-born cases of TB. Blacks or African Americans had the highest number, 43 percent of all U.S.-born cases. Whites have the second-highest burden, representing 33 percent of U.S.-born cases, followed by Hispanics or Latinos (18 percent), Asians (3 percent), American Indians or Alaska Natives (3 percent), and Native Hawaiian or other Pacific Islanders (1 percent). It is important to note that U.S.-born cases of TB represent less than half of the total cases in the United States; 59 percent of all TB cases were among foreign-born persons in 2008.

In 2008, among persons with TB in the United States whose country of origin was known, approximately 95 percent of Asians, 76 percent of Hispanics, 32 percent of blacks, and 18 percent of whites were foreign born. This confirms what we already know—Asia has much higher rates of TB. Consequently, immigrants to the United States from Asia are more likely to have TB than native-born U.S. nationals. According to the World Health Organization, in 2007 the rate of new cases per 100,000 of the population was 98 for China, 171 for Vietnam, and 21 for Japan. These rates are extremely high compared to the rate of 4.2 in the United States. Due to these high rates, Asian origin may be an important risk marker.

Certain risk factors or behaviors contribute to rates among native-born U.S. residents. They include homelessness, incarceration, and a recent history of intravenous drug and alcohol abuse. All these behaviors or factors are common among both U.S.-born blacks and whites who have TB. Education and intervention efforts targeted toward populations at high risk for TB are essential to reach the goal of TB elimination in the United States.

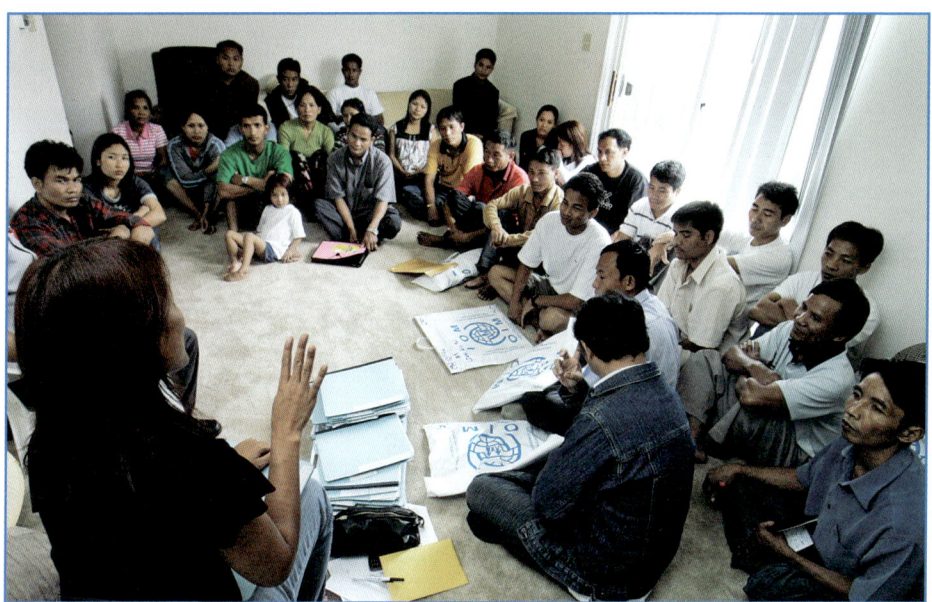

A 2007 flood of refugees from Myanmar, including those shown in the support group above, overwhelmed U.S. aid groups and government services. One chief concern was the threat of the spread of TB, which occurs at a higher rate in Asian countries.

Prison communities are ideal for the spread of TB because prisoners live close together. For example, the incidence of TB among inmates in California state prisons in 1987 was nearly six times that of California's general population. Thus, TB transmission in prisons poses a health problem for the correctional institutions as well as the surrounding communities into which the inmates are released. Consequently, previous incarceration is an important risk factor for TB.

TREATING TB IN THE REST OF THE WORLD

Just as the United States and other developed countries can't stop TB, neither can the rest of the world. In fact, in developing countries, many people are unable to afford any medication.

It has to be provided for free. Who is going to pay for the free medication when poor governments are cash strapped?

Even where free medication is provided, distance keeps some people from getting access to these medications. Such people are more likely to discontinue treatment or take their medicines sporadically. This increases the risk of drug resistance. It also produces disease reservoirs. Unfortunately, such disease reservoirs mean that the world still faces the risk of those diseases.

IS IT POSSIBLE TO ELIMINATE TB IN THE UNITED STATES?

TB in the United States is at its lowest rate since reporting began. Treatment is widely available, and health departments have implemented contact tracing and DOT programs. However, complete elimination of TB in the United States remains an elusive goal. Two main reasons may account for this: the increase of HIV/AIDS in the U.S. population and the increasing influx of immigrants.

HIV/AIDS makes it easy for TB to spread. The weakened immune systems of people living with AIDS make them less able to resist infection. Thus increases in HIV infection mean that more and more people are likely to be infected and develop active TB. Also, the increasing numbers of new arrivals into the United States means that new cases are arriving daily as well. While more stringent screening of immigrants may help, a better solution may be helping to treat TB overseas in the developing countries where treatment facilities are weak and TB care is limited. In fact, without controlling TB in developing countries, control in the United States remains impossible.

Immigrants usually carry the diseases that are dominant in their places of origin. As a result, people originating from areas with high rates of HIV/AIDS or TB are more likely to have those diseases. Even more important, the strains of the disease they carry are more likely the strains circulating in their home regions. Consequently, a foreign-born person with MDR TB most likely originated from an area with high rates of that particular strain of the disease.

Until free TB medication is provided for every person who needs it, it is impossible for the world to rid itself of the disease. The problem is that many people with TB are not aware of their status. The poor health systems in their countries make it difficult to detect and treat disease. That means XDR TB in Afghanistan or Angola puts the whole world at risk.

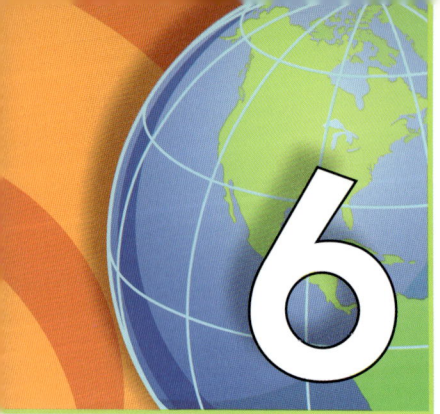

POLIO

For years, children in particular had been paralyzed by a disease caused by the polio virus. Easily spread through human-to-human contact and contaminated food and water, polio spread uncontrollably. That was until the polio vaccine was invented and widely applied. In fact, the vaccine was so successful that in 1988, the World Health Organization expected that polio could be completely eradicated in a few years.

Since then, some 2 billion children have been vaccinated, cutting incidence of the disease more than 99 percent and saving some 5 million children from paralysis or death. But 20 years later, polio is still on the loose in some parts of the world. Total eradication has remained an elusive goal. Cultural suspicions, competition for resources from many other disease afflictions, and simple exhaustion stand in the way. As the polio campaign has shown, even the miracle of discovering a vaccine is not enough. Nevertheless, a massive effort is under way to conquer polio once and for all. The Bill and Melinda Gates Foundation is investing millions into polio eradication.

What is polio? How does it spread? Why has it been so difficult to control? Is there any reason for the renewed optimism? Can the world ever be polio-free? Which parts of the world have seen a polio resurgence and why? These are some of the questions addressed in this chapter. Polio provides a good illustration of the importance of global cooperation against disease. It demonstrates clearly that diseases do not respect political boundaries. Uncontrolled disease in any part of the world puts the entire world at risk.

UNMASKING POLIO

Poliomyelitis (usually called *polio*), a contagious disease, has plagued humans since ancient times. At the height of the polio epidemic in 1952, nearly 60,000 cases with more than 3,000 deaths were reported in the United States alone. Thanks to wide-spread vaccination, polio occurring through natural infection was eliminated from the United States by 1979. But, although it has been eradicated in most developed countries, polio persists in developing countries. Outbreaks are particularly common in Nigeria, Pakistan, and Afghanistan.

Why is it that a disease that has been completely eliminated in large parts of the world continues to pose a serious threat to health elsewhere? What is different in these polio-endemic countries compared to those countries that don't have the disease? What is common among these areas with ongoing polio transmission? Let us begin by learning some fundamentals about the symptoms of polio, the mode of spread, and the challenges of control.

SIGNS AND SYMPTOMS

Polio is a viral illness. It is transmitted mainly through eating or drinking material contaminated with the virus. Infected people usually shed the virus in their feces for several weeks. During that time, polio can spread rapidly in the community. It does so because of poor sanitation habits such as failing to wash your hands after using the bathroom.

The symptoms of polio vary from very mild to very severe. In about 95 percent of cases, it produces no symptoms at all. This is called asymptomatic polio. A more severe form, called paralytic polio, occurs in up to 2 percent of all cases. In such cases, it causes paralysis and can even result in death. Because the virus attacks the nerves that govern the breathing and movement muscles, it causes breathing difficulty and paralysis of the arms and legs. Victims often require crutches, special braces, or even wheelchairs in order to move around.

Polio mainly affects children under five years of age. However, adults can be infected. And when adults do get infected, they carry the virus long enough to spread it from place to place, infecting their close contacts and contaminating sanitation systems. This means that the virus spreads rapidly and easily in areas with poor sanitation systems. In fact, thousands of people may be infected before the first case of polio paralysis emerges. As a result, the WHO considers a single confirmed case of polio paralysis to be evidence of an epidemic.

Eradicating polio means finding ways to get polio drops into the mouth of every child under five years of age—over and over again for several years. It takes many doses to effectively immunize a child. But when the eradication campaign goes on for too long, more than 10 years in some places, exhaustion sets in. The public, the workers, and the government get sick of it. They give up or don't try as hard.

In 1988, when the Global Polio Eradication Initiative began, 355,000 cases of polio were reported in 125 countries. After a few years of the massive oral polio vaccine (OPV) campaign, success was almost at hand. In fact, by the end of 2004, there were just 1,255 cases. But polio refused to be defeated. It bounced back. Between 2002 and 2006, 20 previously polio-free countries in

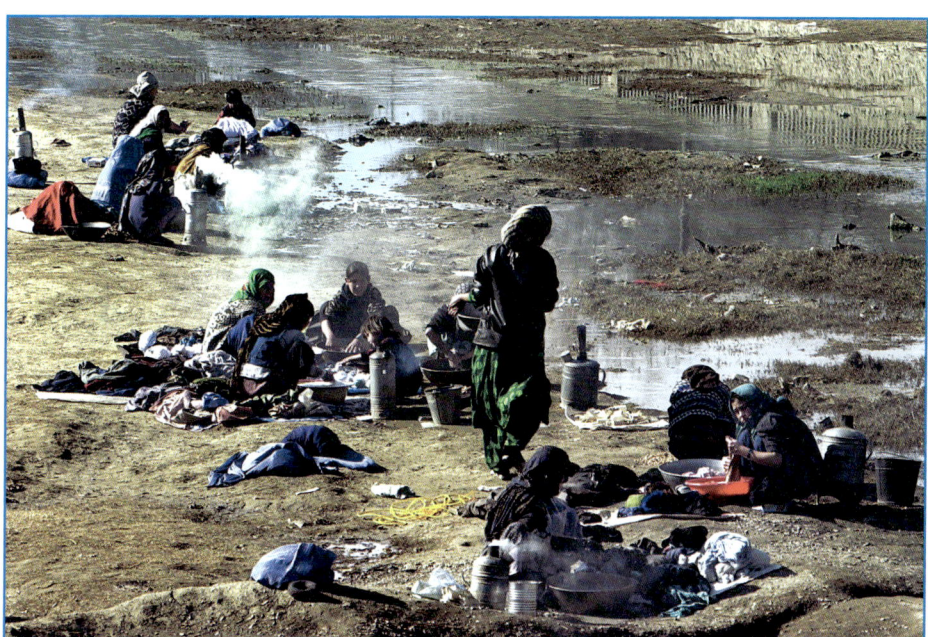

These Afghan women must wash their clothes in a river because they lack an adequate water supply in their homes. Since diseases such as polio are spread through contaminated food and water, areas without proper sanitation are susceptible to rapid transfer of disease.

Africa and Asia reported new cases, all of which originated from Nigeria. By the end of 2007, new cases had stopped in all countries except Angola, Chad, Democratic Republic of the Congo (DRC), Niger, and Sudan.

Once again, during 2008, multiple new cases of ongoing transmission were reported across Africa. In fact, 96 polio cases were reported during January to March 2009 with persistent transmission in five previously polio-free African countries. Like the 2002–2006 resurgence, all of these cases originated from Nigeria or India. Of these, Nigeria was the major source, accounting for 68 polio cases. India was the source of another 28 cases. As of March 24, 2009, multiple outbreaks resulting from importations were ongoing. Three regions of Africa were affected by importations from 2008 to 2009: west central Africa, the Horn of Africa, and south central Africa.

In West Africa, circulation of the polio virus in Nigeria produced importations into eight countries—Benin, Burkina Faso, Chad, Ivory Coast, Ghana, Mali, Niger, and Togo during 2008 and 2009.

The Horn of Africa has seen a series of waves of polio virus outbreaks. In 2003, an importation event originating in Nigeria caused an outbreak of 51 polio cases in Chad. From there it spread to Sudan in mid-2004, resulting in 147 polio cases in that country. Subsequent related transmission occurred in seven other countries (Eritrea, Ethiopia, Indonesia, Kenya, Saudi Arabia, Somalia, and Yemen).

When the Sudan outbreak subsided, no additional cases attributable to the 2004 importation into Sudan were detected until April 2008, after which 53 additional cases were detected: 3 cases in Ethiopia, 2 in northern Kenya, 5 in Uganda, and 43 in Sudan itself. Since 2004, a total of 190 polio cases in Sudan have resulted from the 2004 importation. Another importation into western Sudan occurred in 2008. Originating from Nigeria, it spread through Chad and resulted in two isolated polio cases with no evidence of further spread. Other cases were traceable to previous importations.

In south central Africa, recurrent importation events in Angola, all originating from India, have produced outbreaks. An outbreak in Angola in 2005 ended in 2007 with 19 confirmed cases but led to 58 cases in DRC between 2006 and 2008 and 3 cases in the Central African Republic in 2008. A second importation into Angola originating from northern India was associated with 15 polio cases in Angola during April 2007 to February 2009. Another importation, also originating from northern India, resulted in 24 polio cases in Angola and one case in DRC in 2008. Thus, Angola, Chad, and Sudan have been the source of multiple polio importations to neighboring countries. The countries have also reported their own polio cases since November 2008.

EXPLAINING THE SPATIAL PATTERN

Why is it so difficult to defeat polio in these countries? What cultural practices facilitate polio spread and persistence? Let us explore some reasons.

Poor health resources and war are two main factors. Angola, Chad, Nigeria, and Sudan have very weak health infrastructures. Routine vaccination coverage in certain areas is low. Vaccination efforts don't reach large numbers of children in critical areas because of poor planning and implementation. In addition, Angola, Chad, and Sudan all have experienced civil war in recent years. In fact, Chad and Sudan continued to have civil unrest during 2008 and 2009.

Nigeria was the major reservoir of polio virus for further spread in Africa during 2008 to 2009 and during 2002 to 2006. Polio transmission has never been interrupted in Nigeria. Chronically weak routine vaccination was compounded during 2003 to 2004 by a decrease in vaccine acceptance and an increase of polio spread. During that period, misconceptions about the safety of the vaccine led to loss of public confidence and opposition. As a result, mass immunization efforts in some northern parts of the country were suspended.

Polio control in Nigeria remains a major challenge. From 2002 to 2005, 47 importation events originating from Nigeria affected 16 countries in Africa and resulted in 1,335 polio cases. Nigeria, particularly northern Nigeria, remains a difficult challenge due to ignorance and poor governance. Despite the Nigerian government's efforts, polio vaccines are not effectively reaching children in Kano and several states in northern Nigeria. Between 20 and 30 percent of children in these parts of the country remain unvaccinated.

One problem is that the oral vaccine requires refrigeration in hot temperatures, but refrigerators are rare in these regions. Also, illiteracy and a lack of trust in the government, which is notorious for corruption, are huge problems. In 2003, the vaccination campaign in Kano came to a halt amid rumors that the polio vaccine caused infertility and HIV/AIDS. By the time local leaders became convinced that the rumors were untrue, the virus had "exploded" out of Nigeria. It quickly spread to more than 20 neighboring countries where it had previously been eliminated, as well as to Yemen and distant Indonesia.

Nigerian Muslims going to Saudi Arabia for the annual pilgrimage to Mecca carried the disease with them. And from Mecca, Indonesian Muslims carried the disease home with them. Putting out that fire set the eradication effort back several years and added nearly $1 billion to its cost. More resources would help health workers respond to such a setback in the future, but getting more children to take the vaccines is going to take hard work.

NIGERIA'S POLIO AGONY

In 2004, at the end of the polio vaccine boycott in northern Nigeria, Nigeria's president, Olusegun Obasanjo, apologized for his country's role in reigniting the disease, but the harm was already done. The vaccination campaign had been halted for 10 months. As Kano government officials visited vaccine factories in Indonesia, India, and South Africa, and medical and religious experts from Saudi Arabia flew in to meet local clerics, Kano's governor argued that he had a moral responsibility to stop the vaccination campaign until it was clearly established that there was no harm. His health minister added that Kano residents had become so suspicious of government health workers that they were refusing all vaccinations. Moreover, they couldn't vaccinate people at gunpoint, he said. Opponents of the polio drive claimed that the vaccine was "tainted by evildoers from America" and was "America's revenge for September 11."

Finally, the case was made that the vaccine was safe. In a very public display of support broadcast on national television, Nigeria's president personally gave the polio vaccination drops to a governor's one-year-old daughter in October 2004. That event marked the beginning of a new round of vaccinations for 80 million children.

The new vaccination drive faces extremely difficult challenges. The vaccine must be kept chilled from the time it leaves the factory until it reaches a child's mouth. But in Nigeria, many clinic officials pocket the money provided for buying freezers, leaving the clinics with no freezers. Thus effectiveness of the vaccine is itself an issue.

Finding enough women for the vaccination teams is a particularly tough challenge. Only women can enter a Nigerian Muslim household if the husband is away, and women with children are better at persuading other mothers to vaccinate. But many men refused to let their wives leave home to perform these jobs. They wanted the jobs, which pay about $3 a day, for themselves. That is a huge fortune in a country where most people live on less than $2 a day.

Still, the government seemed determined to succeed. The chief prosecutor of Katsina, another northern Nigerian state, announced that he would jail for a year any parents who refused polio vaccination drops for their children.

DETERMINED TO SAVE OTHERS

Amid all these challenges, there are exciting stories of hope, resilience, and determination. Take the case of Aminu Ahmed. Aminu Ahmed's legs are so withered he must lean on something just to sit up in the cement courtyard of his home in Kano, in northern Nigeria. He "walks" by swinging his hips in an arc on his six-inch hand crutches. He is a victim of polio, but he is a very determined fighter against the disease.

Forty-five years old, Ahmed is the president of the Kano State Polio Victims Association, which owns the welding shop where he builds hand-cranked tricycles for other polio victims. He coached Kano's handicapped soccer team to three national championships. And he owns a home built with money he earned himself. He and his wife, Hadiza, have six children. The youngest, Omar, age two, was born shortly before Kano's government stopped its polio vaccinations. Today, like his father before him, he drags himself across the cement courtyard. The joints of his spindly legs are covered with calluses. He has polio, too.

Ahmed regularly goes on local radio to plead with parents and the government to give their children the polio vaccine. He campaigned aggressively for an end to the vaccination moratorium because he didn't want people to be disabled like him and his son.

IS GLOBAL ERADICATION OF POLIO POSSIBLE?

In the universe of global diseases, polio seems like a minor problem. Fewer than 2,000 people in the world had polio in 2008. AIDS and malaria, by contrast, killed more than 3 million people. Yet, Microsoft's Bill Gates and his foundation gave $255 million to fight polio. In a list of the world's most threatening infectious diseases, polio would rank pretty far down—past measles, meningitis, influenza, and drug-resistant tuberculosis. So why did he give so much money for such an "insignificant" disease?

The answer is that polio is on the brink of being eliminated once and for all. Massive vaccination campaigns around the world, led by the WHO and the Rotary Club International, have reduced cases by 99 percent, leaving only a few isolated pockets of disease. But tracking and inflicting the final blow is a difficult task. The polio virus appears to have established several unassailable strongholds, thanks to cultural misunderstanding, human behavior, and political instability.

An infusion of funds targeted at these remaining strongholds of polio is expected to deliver the knockout blow. Unfortunately, while money is needed, wiping a disease off the face of the planet—especially a disease like polio, which spreads easily and

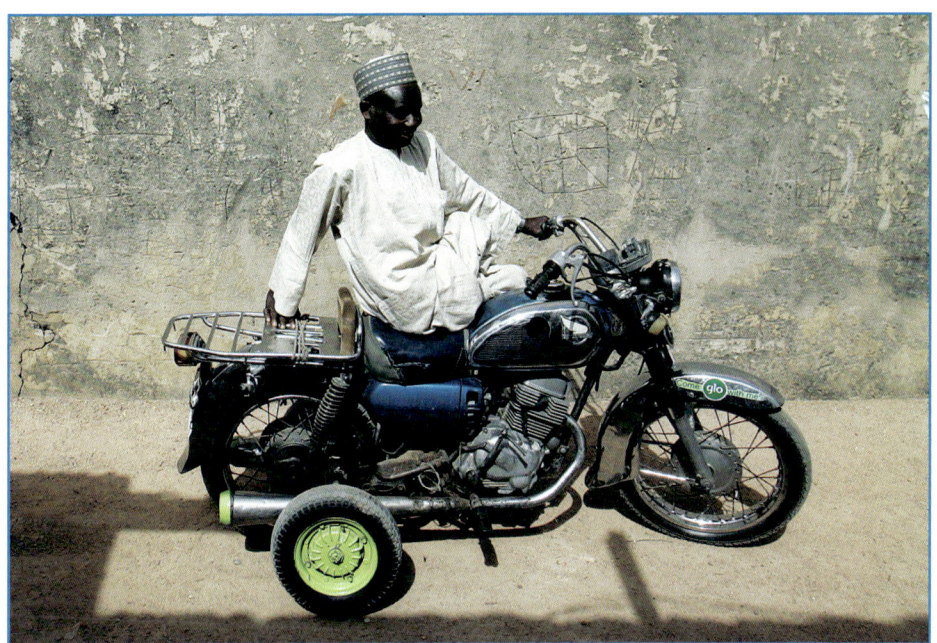

Aminu Ahmed mounts a motorcycle he has modified with side wheels and a hand brake. Since losing the use of his legs to polio, he campaigns tirelessly for the Nigerian government to relent and provide its children with the polio vaccine.

quickly through human-to-human contact and contaminated food and water—is not easy. Because only one in 200 children who contract the virus shows the most visible symptoms of paralysis, the remaining 199 are silent carriers and continue to spread the disease. Indeed, more than two decades of fighting the disease around the globe has taught health workers that it is far more stubborn than originally thought, and the knockout blow will not be easy.

THE CHALLENGE OF POLIO CONTROL IN INDIA

The problems in northern India are completely different but equally difficult. Although the local governments in Uttar

Pradesh and Bihar have been efficient and cooperative in carrying out inoculation, the vaccines themselves are not wholly effective. Scientists don't understand exactly why. But they suspect that the typical child harbors so many intestinal germs that the immune system is overwhelmed and fails to pick up on the vaccine. In relatively sanitary Europe or the United States,

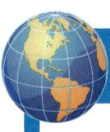

MAKING C⬤NNECTI⬤NS

CONQUERING SMALLPOX—
THE MASSIVE KILLER DISEASE

Smallpox, an acute contagious disease caused by a virus, originated more than 3,000 years ago in India or Egypt. One of the most devastating diseases known to humanity, its repeated epidemics swept across continents, decimating populations for centuries. In some ancient cultures, smallpox was such a major killer of infants that newborns were not named until they had caught the disease and proved they would survive.

Smallpox devastation was extensive. It killed as many as 30 percent of those infected, but between 65 and 80 percent of survivors were marked with deep, pitted scars on the face. Blindness was another complication. In eighteenth-century Europe, one-third of all reported cases of blindness were due to smallpox. At that time, smallpox killed every tenth child born in Sweden and France and every seventh child born in Russia. In Vietnam in 1898, 95 percent of adolescent children were pockmarked, and nine-tenths of all blindness was due to smallpox.

The disease did not discriminate based on age, wealth, or even fame. Famous world leaders killed by smallpox include Queen Mary II of England, Emperor Joseph I of Austria, King Luis I of Spain, Tsar Peter II of Russia, Queen Ulrika Elenora of Sweden, and King Louis XV of France.

a child typically requires three doses of an oral vaccine to gain immunity; in northern India, a child needs as many as 12 doses. Getting this medicine to children and keeping track of those who have received it is a staggering challenge.

New funding would help, of course. Contributions from the Bill and Melinda Gates Foundation, the Rotary Club International,

Edward Jenner discovered a vaccine in 1798. This brought the first hope that the disease could be controlled. In the early 1950s—150 years after the introduction of vaccination—an estimated 50 million cases of smallpox occurred in the world each year. By the end of 1966, vaccination had cut this figure drastically to around 10 million to 15 million.

In 1967, smallpox threatened 60 percent of the world's population. It killed every fourth victim and scarred or blinded most survivors. In that year, the WHO launched an intensified effort to eradicate the disease. Through this massive global effort, smallpox was finally conquered. The last natural case occurred in Somalia in 1977. Global eradication was completed and certified by the World Health Assembly in 1980.

Smallpox eradication was a global campaign. Populations were protected by vaccination in every country. Since then, immunization has stopped in many countries. In the United States, smallpox vaccination ended in 1972. In 1979, the WHO recommended that vaccination against smallpox be stopped in all countries, except among special groups, such as researchers working with smallpox and related viruses. By 1986, routine vaccination had ceased in all countries.

But are we completely safe? Data from the eradication campaign show that immunity wanes with time. Could smallpox come back again? What would happen if it did?

and the German and British governments amount to about $630 million toward the effort. This can help bring injectable vaccines, which are more effective and expensive than the oral versions, to India. It could also help to expand campaigns in Nigeria, reaching more children and increasing the presence of health workers to advocate for the program.

However, it may not do much in war-torn countries such as Pakistan and Afghanistan, where the disease thrives and violence and war impede prevention efforts. Water lines and sanitation facilities will not be built when bombs are exploding everywhere and bullets are flying overhead. New funding is absolutely necessary but may not be sufficient to eradicate the disease. It all depends on what happens in the countries and at local levels, especially in the rural areas. Will the world stop war and deal with diseases that are killing children?

POLIO IN PAKISTAN

Pakistan is another country with recurrent polio outbreaks. Parts of the country are experiencing conflict, even war. Cultural obstacles are also preventing efforts. All of these make polio control in Pakistan a steep uphill battle. These problems are compounded by a huge problem of poor health infrastructure and weak surveillance systems.

Cultural beliefs and obstacles are a huge problem in Pakistan. For example, several parents refused to get their children vaccinated against polio. Thus, many children are not getting the full or required dosage of the vaccine. In a recent case, a nine-month-old boy had received seven doses of polio vaccination drops during special campaigns, but he did not get vaccinated during routine immunization. His mother refused to allow him to be vaccinated.

What should be done in such a situation? Should the mother be compelled to vaccinate that child? Should the WHO take the child away from the mother and forcibly vaccinate him or her?

Remember that as long as one person remains unvaccinated, polio remains a threat.

Let us personalize this. If you were the parent and the government or some health authority figure came and told you to have your child immunized, how would you react? Is it okay for the child to be immunized against the wishes of the parent? What about nations? Should Nigeria be forced to implement more thorough polio vaccinations? Even more basic, should countries be forced or required to report all internal disease outbreaks and not conceal them? What sanctions can be brought against those nations or people who refuse to comply?

Insecurity

Another problem in Pakistan is insecurity, especially war. Health workers attribute the recent rise in the number of cases to the fighting between the Pakistani army and Islamist militants. During active conflict, health workers are unable to go to those areas for immunization exercises. For nearly a year, it was impossible to continue the immunization exercise due to the security situation. Meanwhile, war and bombs are unable to stop the polio virus from spreading. Sadly, as the bullets fly, roadside bombs go off, and health workers run for cover, polio marches on. And children remain victims, fodder for the disease.

As in Nigeria, another obstacle is the low proportion of female teams. Islamic Pakistani culture has stringent laws about gender spatial segregation. Only women can enter a Muslim household if the husband is away, and women with children are better at persuading other mothers to vaccinate their children. Variable routine immunization coverage, pockets of refusals in a few key districts, rapid turnover of district health leaderships, and low public demand for immunization are also important impediments. Poor sanitation and high population density, which lead to a high prevalence of diarrheal disease, also interfere with the uptake of the oral polio vaccine in the intestines of children. All these factors have hampered the eradication efforts.

Refusals

Refusal is a significant problem in a few districts of Pakistan, including Killa Abdullah, Bajaur, Mohamand, and Swat. Overall, less than one percent of the targeted children are missed because of refusals, so it cannot be the main cause of the resurgence of polio cases. Some attribute it to polio campaign fatigue, noting that some houses had been missed during house-to-house calls. The problem is that new polio cases were not only arising in inaccessible areas. The disease was widespread.

ASMA—PARALYZED BY POLIO IN PAKISTAN

Nine-month-old Asma was a healthy little girl until she suddenly fell ill with a high fever in May 2003. At a nearby rural health center, examination and tests confirmed that she had contracted polio. Her left leg was paralyzed, and even today, Asma can't stand without support.

Asma was one of the unfortunate seven confirmed cases of polio in Thatta, a village in Pakistan. The other six confirmed cases included four girls and three boys. Despite the serious nature of the polio outbreak, local residents were reluctant to have their children vaccinated. Parents, religious leaders, teachers, and health workers were all disinterested and tired of the polio vaccination campaign.

That is when UNICEF stepped in. To eradicate polio and protect children in Thatta and elsewhere in Pakistan, UNICEF embarked on a massive campaign. More than 560 mobile vaccination teams traveled by foot, bicycle, and motorbike to reach 220,000 children under the age of five living in sparsely populated settlements spread across the district's vast and barren land. In addition, 85 health posts were set up for routine immunization, and another 32 transit points were built to track children who were missed in the campaigns.

In one instance, a community leader refused to allow the vaccinators access to his area. He had read a newspaper report that claimed that the polio vaccine was ineffective, he said. The vaccination team

Finding Creative Ways to Fight Polio

Pakistan has employed some very creative ways to continue the fight against polio. One of them, the polio bicycle campaign, was an unusual kind of rally that conveyed a powerful message. Twelve boys paralyzed by polio were on their wheelchairs at the front of a bicycle rally organized by the Balochistan Boy Scouts Association in the capital of the Balochistan province in West Pakistan. Their objective was to raise public awareness about polio and the urgency to drive the disease from Pakistan. More

leader met and tried to persuade him, but he would not budge. Finally in desperation, in front of the community leader and all the villagers, the team leader gave polio drops to his own son. The technique worked well, and the door was opened for the vaccination effort.

Since 2003, Pakistan has made remarkable progress in eliminating polio. During each immunization round, nearly 32 million children under age five have received the oral polio vaccine. In 2004, the number of polio cases was reduced to 53. But Pakistan still remains polio endemic and a huge concern for the rest of the world. Eradicating polio locally is a crucial step in stopping polio transmission globally. But security concerns remain a major obstacle. In areas such as North-West Frontier Province/Federally Administered Tribal Areas (FATA), security concerns and the associated large-scale population movements make it difficult to reach immunization targets.

There are some hopeful signs, however. In February 2009, Pakistan's prime minister, Yousuf Raza Gilani, launched a Polio Action Plan, with the immediate aim of providing high-level support for polio eradication and fostering provincial- and district-level accountability and cooperation. While these efforts are encouraging, for little Asma, they come too late. She is already paralyzed and will remain that way the rest of her life.

than 12 million children were targeted to be immunized against polio in this campaign as part of Pakistan's efforts to eradicate the disease. This campaign was critically important because it was taking place in the high-risk districts of the country.

Campaigns are reaching a vast majority of the children under age five. About 97 percent of children were vaccinated in Quetta in a previous campaign, while 95 percent of children were reached in Killa Abdullah, a district in northern Balochistan where some families reject the vaccine due to misconceptions. But still it is vital to reach every child under five during each round. Only then can polio finally be eradicated from Pakistan.

Schoolchildren are helping, too. Two girls, Shakila, 15, and Nasra, 16, support the campaign as vaccinators in their mixed Christian and Muslim neighborhood. They are one key to the successful reach of the program in Pakistan. Female teams get unhindered access to households. This is Shakila's eighth campaign. When she finishes her studies, she would like to be a paramedic, also known in Pakistan as a "lady health worker." Nasra would like to become a teacher. The girls know the area well, and practically all the parents let them vaccinate their children. For their work, they receive 150 Pakistani rupees (about $2.50) per day.

Polio campaigns in Pakistan face immense challenges. The teams of vaccinators have three days to reach every child under five in the communities and two days more to address the refusals and vaccinate the children who missed the polio drops. Reaching nomad populations and refugees is also a challenge.

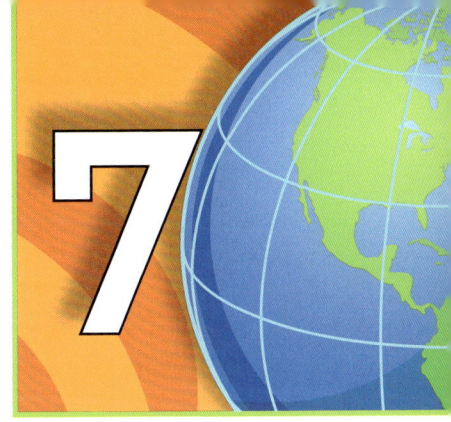

THE COMING
PANDEMICS?

In 2009, fear of another global pandemic gripped the world. This time it was H1N1, more commonly known as swine flu. In the United States, schools were closed and hospital emergency rooms were flooded with people complaining of respiratory symptoms. In Mexico, the supposed origin of the disease, the entire nation came to an almost total shutdown as schools, restaurants, government buildings, and even stadiums were closed for about one week. In Egypt, all the pigs were slaughtered. China quarantined some 200 people in a hotel with armed guards because they had arrived in the country on the same flight as a man who had flu symptoms.

Yet all these efforts could not stop swine flu. The disease marched on. In June 2009, it was wreaking havoc in the Southern Hemisphere in places like Australia and Argentina. In the Northern Hemisphere, in countries like the United States and Canada, people feared the worst—a winter return of swine flu with a vengeance!

Before swine flu, there was avian influenza. Caused by human contact with birds carrying the virus, it killed 60 percent of infected people. As it spread over the world, the panic was global. What if it mutated to become human-to-human transmissible? But then, it fizzled away. Prior to avian influenza, there was SARS. Easily transmitted between humans, it was killing 10 percent of those infected.

SARS

Severe acute respiratory syndrome (SARS) is a serious form of pneumonia. It is caused by a virus that was isolated for the first time in 2003. Infection with the SARS virus results in severe breathing difficulty and sometimes death. This contagious respiratory infection was first described in February 2003. Dr. Carlo Urbani, a World Health Organization physician, diagnosed the first case of SARS. It was carried by a 48-year-old businessman who had traveled from the Guangdong province of China, through Hong Kong, to Hanoi, Vietnam. The businessman died from the illness. About a month later, Dr. Urbani died from the disease at the age of 46.

Within six weeks of its discovery, SARS had infected thousands of people around the world, including people in Asia, Australia, Europe, Africa, and North and South America. Schools were closed throughout Hong Kong and Singapore. National economies were affected. By the time it was over, more than 8,439 people had been sickened with the disease and 812 had died in 30 different countries. Places that were closely linked by international travel suffered the most from SARS.

SARS arrived in North America through Canada. A Canadian family of Hong Kong descent who lived in Toronto became the first cases. During their travel to Hong Kong, the 78-year-old woman and her husband stayed at a hotel where 13 people were later confirmed to have the disease. Two days after returning home, the woman developed what is now known as SARS and died. Several of her close family members then developed SARS symptoms. One of them was admitted to a hospital that became the center of the Toronto outbreak. SARS killed 44 Canadians and made hundreds of people sick. More than 25,000 residents of the Greater Toronto area were put in quarantine to prevent further spread of the disease.

The WHO identified SARS as a global health threat and issued an unprecedented travel advisory. Daily WHO updates tracked the spread of SARS seven days a week. The rapid, global public health response helped to stem the spread of the virus. And by June 2003, the epidemic had subsided to the degree that on June 7 the WHO backed off from its daily reports. Nevertheless, even as the number of new cases dwindled and travel advisories began to be lifted, the sober truth remained: Every new case had the potential to spark another outbreak. SARS appears to be here to stay and to have changed the way that the world responds to infectious diseases in the era of widespread international travel. SARS showed very dramatically how quickly world travel can spread a disease and also how quickly global networking and cooperation can respond to an emerging threat.

H5N1 AVIAN INFLUENZA

Just as the world was beginning to breathe a sigh of relief from SARS, avian influenza appeared. The threat of an influenza pandemic immediately triggered alarm around the world. It was extremely contagious, spread by coughing and sneezing, and easily transmissible. If a fully transmissible pandemic virus emerged, the spread of the disease could not be prevented. Pandemic influenza would have devastating consequences. Experience with past pandemics suggested that more than 1.5 billion people could be sickened. Even if the virus caused relatively mild disease, the economic and social disruption arising from sudden surges of illness in so many people would be enormous. As news headlines warned of pandemic influenza that could kill 150 million people, the world sprang into action. Millions of chickens and domestic birds were killed, and avian influenza subsided for a while.

Avian influenza is caused by a virus that occurs naturally among wild birds. Although the birds shed the virus in their saliva and feces, they usually do not get sick from it. However, domestic birds such as chickens, ducks, and turkeys become infected through contact with birds that carry the virus. People who have contact with infected birds or contaminated surfaces get the infection, but human-to-human spread of avian influenza is rare. Symptoms of avian influenza in humans include fever, cough, sore throat, muscle aches, eye infections, and severe breathing problems.

Between 2003 and 2009, the World Health Organization reported 417 cases of H5N1, with 257 deaths (see Table 7.1). That means H5N1 killed about 6 out of every 10 infected people. However, the death rate was very different among countries. With 141 cases and 115 deaths, Indonesia was the most severely affected country. More than 80 percent of the cases died there. Vietnam was the second most severely affected country. Half of the 110 people infected with the disease died. Egypt had 63 cases with 23 deaths, but 25 of China's 38 cases died. Clearly, H5N1 was more deadly in some places than others. In Nigeria, Africa's most populous country, only one case was reported, with one death. Can you give some reasons for these differences? Perhaps quality of health care available is one reason. Can you think of any other reasons?

Avian influenza was not as deadly as feared. But the disease has not gone away. Nor has it become less lethal or less widespread in birds. Experts argue that preparations against it have to continue. Its failure to mutate into a pandemic strain has given the world more breathing room. There were 86 confirmed human cases in 2007 compared with 115 in 2006, according to the World Health Organization, and 59 deaths compared with 79. Experts assume that the real numbers are several times larger because many cases are missed.

TABLE 7.1 TOTAL H5N1 CASES AND DEATHS REPORTED TO WHO 2003–2009			
Country	Total Cases	Total Deaths	%
Azerbaijan	8	5	62.5
Bangladesh	1	0	0.0
Cambodia	8	7	87.5
China	38	25	65.8
Djibouti	1	0	0.0
Egypt	63	23	36.5
Indonesia	141	115	81.6
Iraq	3	2	66.7
Laos	2	2	100.0
Myanmar	1	0	0.0
Nigeria	1	1	100.0
Pakistan	3	1	33.3
Thailand	25	17	68.0
Turkey	12	4	33.3
Vietnam	110	55	50.0
Total	417	257	61.6
Source: WHO, 2009			

Despite the culling of hundreds of millions of birds and the injection of billions of doses of poultry vaccine, the virus remained out of control in some of the most populous countries, though exactly which ones are in dispute. In Egypt, Indonesia, and Nigeria, it remained endemic in local birds. Reports of recurrent outbreaks persisted in parts of India, Myanmar, and Pakistan. Villagers in India were reported to be killing and eating their flocks before government cullers, who paid less than a third of market value, could seize them.

One positive effect of the scare of avian influenza was increased global pandemic preparedness. Vaccines were developed. Stockpiles of Tamiflu and masks were ready. Many countries, cities, companies, and schools wrote pandemic plans. In the worst-hit countries laboratories have become faster at flu tests. Government veterinarians now move more quickly to cull chickens. And there is much greater global cooperation and collaboration to fight disease.

But faster vaccine preparation methods are needed. Using current technology, it takes six to eight months to produce a vaccine. It will take a year to produce a billion doses of any vaccine based on a new pandemic strain. But the pandemic would have circled the globe within three months.

SWINE FLU: H1N1

The world got a major scare in April 2009 with the Mexican swine flu outbreak. In days, the disease spread to several states in the United States as well as European countries. Mexico closed all schools—an almost total nationwide shutdown—for five days. Soccer stadiums were empty, even when the most popular teams were playing. Police officers were distributing masks.

Swine flu was declared a global pandemic on June 11, 2009, in the first designation by the World Health Organization of a worldwide pandemic in 41 years. What is swine flu? How do you get it? Where did it come from? How does it spread? Which countries have been most severely affected and why? These are the questions we answer in this section.

Swine flu A (H1N1) is a respiratory disease. Like the seasonal flu, it is spread through the air and also by touching a surface with the virus on it and then touching one's mouth or nose. Frequent hand washing and avoiding surfaces that might be contaminated are wise precautions. This is important because most people lack immunity to this new virus.

However, it appears that influenza A (H1N1) is only slightly more contagious than the seasonal flu. Each infected person is, on average, passing the disease along to between 1.4 and 1.8 people. It is unclear how deadly H1N1 will be. The seasonal flu kills an estimated 250,000 to 500,000 people worldwide each year—36,000 in the United States alone. This outbreak has caused concern because officials have never seen this particular strain of the flu passing among humans before.

One concern is the age of swine flu victims. Unlike typical flu seasons, when infants and the aged are the most vulnerable, the swine flu appears to infect an unusually high percentage of young people. The median age of patients is 17. Pandemic influenza, such as the 1918 flu and outbreaks in 1957 and 1968, often strikes young, healthy people the hardest.

Tracing the Origin of H1N1

Where and how it all began remains a medical mystery. One of the first hints of trouble appeared toward the end of winter, just when the flu season should be ending. It came from the Mexican state of Veracruz—a region that supplies Mexico with much of its pork products from the many villages with pig-breeding factory farms. People in the region have long complained that the huge lagoons of pig waste have contaminated their groundwater. They are frustrated and angry about the stench and the swarms of flies that invade their villages. La Gloria, a hillside hamlet (population 3,000) where people started complaining of bad colds at the end of February 2009, is one of these pig-breeding towns.

On March 23, 2009, Veracruz health officials arrived to take saliva samples. About a third of some 1,300 townspeople who sought medical attention were diagnosed with acute respiratory infections and given surgical masks and antibiotics. Edgar Hernandez lives in La Gloria. He fell ill a bit later; the energetic 5-year-old retreated to his bed with a high fever. Other kids in his school were already sick. A week after his illness, Mexican health authorities confirmed that Edgar was infected with a new

H1N1 influenza strain—a hybrid of pig, bird, and human flu virus. Two children from La Gloria died before being tested; their parents refused to let them be exhumed.

Whether La Gloria is ground zero in this outbreak is not yet known. Mexican health officials dispute this. But by early April, the Veracruz government notified Mexican authorities of a possible flu outbreak in La Gloria. This alert happened to come around Holy Week, a time when most people in this largely Catholic country travel to visit family. On April 12, Mexican health authorities notified the CDC and the Pan American Health Organization of the unexplained cases of severe respiratory illness.

The following day, people started dying. As much of Mexico shut down in panic, cases began to emerge in New York City, the southwestern United States, and around the world. By early May 2009, swine flu had spread so widely that it had become a global disease. The World Health Organization declared it a global pandemic on June 11, 2009.

How Mexico Dealt with the Swine Flu

Mexico decreed an almost total nationwide shutdown for five days. With all schools closed, parents had a huge challenge on their hands. Keeping their kids at home and away from disease while not going crazy themselves wasn't easy. Mexico's traditional cultural practices of kissing, hugging, handshakes, eating on the street, and congregating in public places were all discouraged.

In obedience to government orders, Mexicans locked themselves inside in fear of the virus. By the millions they donned surgical masks, and these became canvases for creativity. Masks were decorated with painted-on monkey mouths, outsized mustaches, or "kissy lips." Newspapers offered smiley cutouts for people to paste on their masks, and some drivers fashioned masks for their cars. Dog lovers walked the streets of Mexico City with matching masks for their pooches.

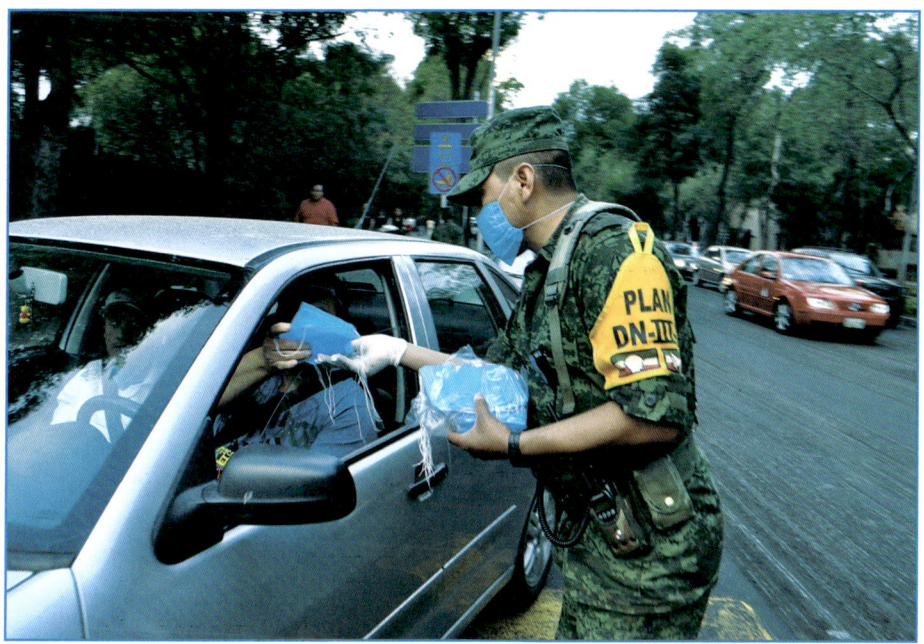

A Mexican soldier distributes surgical masks at an intersection in Mexico City in April 2009. The swine flu (H1N1) began in Mexico, and within days it had spread to other countries.

With no place for people to go, television became one of the only available distractions. But even here, swine flu made its mark on that most Mexican form of entertainment: the soap opera. Nothing defines Mexican soap operas more than overly dramatic kisses. But to accommodate swine flu, Televisa, the world's biggest producer of the soaps, decreed that smooching should be reduced to a minimum in accordance with government guidelines to avoid close contact. Passionate kisses were replaced by air-blown kisses.

Many Mexicans responded to swine flu with humor. They called the disease "the Aporkalypse." "Did you hear that Mexico has become a world power?" goes one joke. "When it sneezes, the whole world gets the flu."

Interestingly, the dark humor spread beyond Mexico's borders, just like swine flu. A U.S. company rolled out T-shirts featuring a pig-shaped Mexican flag. "I went to Mexico and all I got was swine flu," it reads. Swine flu Facebook pages emerged. By April 26, the most popular—set up with a profile picture of a cute white pig—had accumulated more than 20,000 fans.

Swine Flu in the United States

By the end of June 2009, swine flu had infected more than a million Americans and was infecting thousands more every week even though the annual flu season was well over. Because of the difficulty of counting, most experts believe that this number is an underestimate. Moreover, only a tiny fraction of those million cases have been tested. The flu had spread all over the country. There were outbreaks in 34 summer camps in 16 states. About 3,000 Americans had been hospitalized. Of those, 127 had died. The median age of these victims was just 19.

In the early days of the swine flu outbreak in the United States, the cases were concentrated in New York City. Some of the first reported cases were diagnosed in late April 2009 among teenagers from a high school in Queens who had traveled to Mexico for spring break. In the following weeks, New York's public schools seemed to become an incubator for the flu, and numerous facilities were closed. The New York School for Autistic Children was affected and closed down. Emergency personnel wearing masks were seen in front of Public School 177, a school for autistic children, in Queens. Mayor Michael Bloomberg said that 82 of 380 students at the school for autistic children had called in sick.

Initial reaction in the United States was characterized by extreme caution. Many schools were closed. A United Airlines flight from Germany heading to Washington, D.C., was diverted to Boston because a passenger complained of flu-like symptoms. After the woman was checked at Massachusetts General Hospital, the flight continued to Washington Dulles International airport. The airline says the pilot landed in Boston on the advice of the CDC. The flight had 245 passengers and 14 crew members.

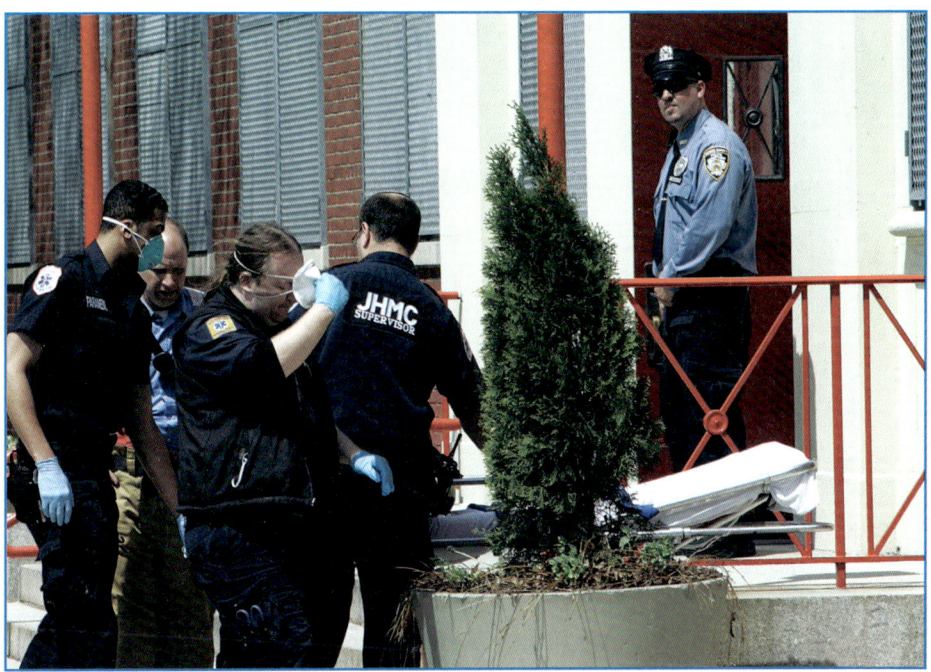

Emergency personnel push a stretcher into Public School 177, a school for autistic children, in New York City in April 2009. Some of the first cases of swine flu reported in the United States were by Queens teenagers who had recently traveled to Mexico.

Most of the initial U.S. cases were traced to Mexico. Take the story of 9-year-old George. He arrived at a medical clinic in Elyria, Ohio, an industrial city 20 miles (32 kilometers) southwest of Cleveland. He had a sore throat, body aches, fever, and dizziness. The pediatric nurse practitioner said it was probably strep throat or an allergy. George's mother mentioned to the nurse that they had just returned from visiting relatives in Mexico. She didn't think it was swine flu because no one else in the family was sick. But it was.

On her way to work that morning, the nurse had heard a radio news report about swine flu turning up in states bordering

Mexico. Although Ohio is far away from Mexico, she wondered if swine flu could spread to their part of the country. After a rapid strep test on the boy came back negative, the nurse did a nasal swab. A half hour later, the lab called to report that George had a type of influenza linked to swine flu virus. Later, the CDC confirmed that the third-grader from Ohio had swine flu. Swine flu had traveled to Ohio through George.

The first recorded swine flu death on U.S. soil was a Mexican toddler who died in Houston, Texas, where the family was seeking health care. In mid-May, an assistant principal at a school in Queens, New York, became the first person to die from the virus in New York. Health officials said that he had a history of medical problems that may have put him at greater risk. Most of those who have died from swine flu in the United States had some underlying condition such as morbid obesity, pregnancy, asthma, diabetes, or immune system problems. They were usually relatively young.

By the first week of July 2009, swine flu was the predominant flu type circulating in the United States. Ten states had reported widespread cases: California, Connecticut, Delaware, Georgia, Hawaii, Maine, New York, Pennsylvania, Rhode Island, and Virginia.

Global Reactions to Swine Flu

The reaction to swine flu across the world was similar and yet different—panic, caution, humor, and acceptance. Here are a few examples.

Argentina

With at least 43 fatalities, Argentina surged into third place in the world for swine flu deaths by the end of June 2009, tailing only Mexico and the United States. Argentina had at least 1,580 confirmed cases of the illness. In contrast, Brazil and Chile, whose epidemics started at roughly the same time, had only one and 14 deaths, respectively.

Health officials said the worsening situation in Argentina, where the Southern Hemisphere winter was just beginning, serves as a warning about the potential for swine flu to spread quickly with colder temperatures. It also emphasizes the need for careful pandemic planning.

Argentina has very little capacity to deal with swine flu. In June 2009, emergency rooms that normally receive 200 patients a day had to attend to 1,000. In Buenos Aires Province, the minister of health said about 40 percent of health care workers were not showing up, either because they were ill or were concerned about catching the virus. The province had called up retired doctors and medical students to help out.

Another problem was the shortage of antiviral drugs. Patients with serious symptoms need to be put on Tamiflu within the first 48 hours. But Argentina, with a population of 40 million, had a stockpile of just about 2 million courses of antiviral drugs. Thus, distribution could be a serious problem. For comparison, the United States, with a population some seven times larger, had 50 million courses of treatment in its Strategic National Stockpile when the pandemic began.

Neighboring Chile had been administering Tamiflu in all suspected cases to contain the virus. This is probably one reason that Chile has seen fewer swine flu deaths. Unfortunately, Argentina did not have enough of the drug to do that. Argentina reported its first confirmed case of swine flu on May 7—an Argentine tourist who returned from Mexico in April.

Egypt

In Egypt, the government ordered the slaughter of the roughly 300,000 pigs in the country in the spring of 2009. That surely was an extreme move since no cases of swine flu had been reported in the country. But the government presented it as a precaution against swine flu. Infuriated, farmers resisted the move and demanded compensation. But the government's action makes sense when put in historical context.

Egypt was among the countries hardest hit by avian influenza. As we have already seen, it had the world's fourth-highest death toll—after Indonesia, Vietnam, and China—and the largest outside of Asia. The WHO confirmed 23 deaths in Egypt.

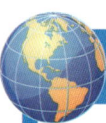

MAKING C⊕NNECTI⊕NS

WHERE IS THE PIG THAT STARTED THE SWINE FLU?

Contrary to the popular assumption that the new swine flu pandemic arose on factory farms in Mexico, researchers now believe that it most likely emerged in pigs in Asia. From there, it traveled to North America in a human. But there is no way to prove their theory. They say that while there is no evidence that this new virus, which combines Eurasian and North American genes, has ever circulated in North American pigs, there is evidence that a closely related "sister virus" has circulated in Asia.

Here is the hypothesis. American breeding pigs, possibly carrying North American swine flu, are frequently exported to Asia, where the flu could have combined with Asian strains. But because disease quarantines make it hard to import Asian pigs, it is unlikely that a pig brought the new strain back to North America. The most likely scenario is that it came over through humans, who move freely around the world. The first person to carry the flu to North America from Asia, assuming that is what happened, has never been found. And he or she will never be discovered because people stop carrying the virus when they get better.

The current swine flu virus sweeping around the world is highly unusual. It includes genetic bits of human, avian, and swine flu from North America as well as Eurasian swine flu. It has not been detected in any pigs except those in a single herd in Canada that was found

Before avian influenza, chickens used to roam the dusty streets in the villages and the city alleys of Egypt. But when avian influenza first appeared there in February 2006, 25 million birds were killed within weeks, devastating the poultry industry and par-

infected in late April 2009. A carpenter who worked on the farm after visiting Mexico had been thought to have infected the herd. But in mid-June, after considerable tests, Canadian health authorities said he was not to blame. The whole herd was culled, and the virus has not been found in any pigs elsewhere in Canada.

However, a sample taken from a pig in Hong Kong in 2004 was recently found to have a virus nearly matching the new swine flu. Because that flu had seven of the new flu's eight genome sequences, an article in *Nature* magazine on June 11, 2009, called it a sister virus. Unfortunately, because there is very little data on swine flu gene sequences from Asia and virtually none from South America or Africa, it is impossible to confirm this.

The new virus was first isolated in late April by American and Canadian laboratories from samples taken from people with flu in Mexico, Southern California, and Texas. The earliest known human case was traced to a 5-year-old boy in La Gloria, a rural town in Veracruz, Mexico. Because that area has many hog-fattening operations with thousands of pigs in crowded barns near lagoons of manure, opponents of factory farming blame the industry. But tests of the pigs on the Veracruz farms by Mexican officials found them free of the virus.

We may never find the pig that brought us swine flu. But if this theory is true, then swine flu is truly the product of globalization—globalized food production and supply and unrestricted rapid global travel. In a globalized world, global pandemics appear to be inevitable.

ticularly the family farmers. Chickens vanished from sight, having been slaughtered, abandoned, or locked away by a population increasingly aware of, and frightened by, the disease's stubborn grip. The swine flu prevention measure appeared designed to avert a similar panic. Yet swine flu continues to move through Egypt.

Australia

Australian authorities told parents not to panic after the country announced its first child death linked to swine flu. By the first week of July 2009, 10 people had died from the virus. As panic set in, the health minister tried to assure people that the virus was mild in most cases. Later that same month, Australia was the worst-hit nation in the Asia-Pacific region, with 4,568 cases.

The government was most concerned about a possible outbreak among Aborigines. This is because Aborigines have poor health status that puts them at increased risk for swine flu. They are more likely to be malnourished and poor, with higher rates of most diseases. Risk behaviors such as tobacco and alcohol use, drug abuse, physical inactivity, and low intake of fruit and vegetables are also widespread in the Aboriginal community.

Aboriginal children often experience poor living conditions; diarrheal diseases and respiratory infections are also common. Vaccine-preventable diseases such as measles, mumps, diphtheria, and tetanus are also rife. All of these make the Aboriginal population of Australia a particularly vulnerable group for swine flu. One Aboriginal man had already died from swine flu by July 1, 2009.

The United Kingdom

In the United Kingdom, the government declared that the rising numbers of swine flu cases made trying to contain the virus no longer an option. In the first week of July 2009, the government was preparing to see about 100,000 new cases each day. That meant anti-flu drugs were no longer available for close contacts of those infected but had to be reserved for confirmed cases. To relieve the pressure on the health service, lab testing to confirm cases was also discontinued.

If doctors believed a person was suffering from swine flu, he or she was told to stay at home and was given a voucher that a friend or family member could take to a drug collection point, such as a pharmacy. Several schools were closed. The United Kingdom had more than 7,000 confirmed cases by the first week of July, and most people thought that was a gross underestimate. Three people had died, but all had underlying health problems.

What's Next, Swine Flu?

Swine flu has sickened hundreds of people all over the world from New York to New Zealand, including children, teens, adults, students, and tourists. It has rattled the world's financial markets, pushed oil prices down, caused a run on surgical masks and hand sanitizers, closed schools and churches, and postponed sporting events. No one knows precisely where the swine flu virus will pop up next. All we know is that it will. Political boundaries can't keep it out.

Globalization has made it easier for swine flu to spread around the world. Because of extensive global travel, no country is safe from the diseases that exist in other countries. Global cooperation is needed to limit or control these diseases. Poor, developing countries usually lack the resources needed to track newly emerging or re-emerging diseases before they spread worldwide. This means that Americans and Canadians may have excellent health care systems, but they are at risk of communicable diseases that break out in Mexico or even in the remotest parts of Afghanistan.

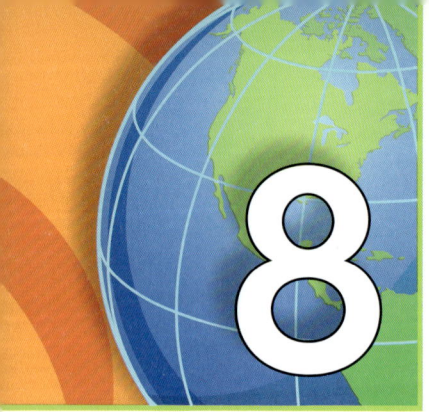

EMERGING AND REEMERGING PANDEMICS

Fifty years ago, many people believed that the age-old battle of humans against infectious disease was virtually over, with humankind the winner. The events of the past two decades have shown the error of that position. At least a dozen "new" diseases have been identified (including AIDS). And traditional diseases that appeared to be on their way out (such as malaria and tuberculosis) are resurging. Globally, infectious diseases remain the leading cause of death, and they are the third-leading cause of death in the United States. Clearly, the battle has not been won.

EMERGING INFECTIOUS DISEASES

Before we go further we need to clarify some terms. *Emerging diseases* are diseases that:

(1) have not occurred in humans before (this is probably rare and difficult to establish);

(2) have occurred previously but affected only small numbers of people in isolated places (AIDS and Ebola hemorrhagic fever are examples); or

(3) have occurred throughout human history but have only recently been recognized as distinct diseases due to an infectious agent. Lyme disease and gastric ulcers are examples.

Environmental changes are related to the emergence of many infectious diseases. For example, Lyme disease emerged when large numbers of people began encountering the insect vector, the deer tick, in greater numbers than ever before.

Reemerging infectious diseases are diseases that were once major health problems globally or in a particular country. They declined dramatically but are again becoming health problems for a significant proportion of the population. Malaria and tuberculosis are excellent examples.

Tuberculosis has reemerged because the pathogen has acquired resistance to the antibiotics used. Malaria has also become drug resistant, and the vector mosquito has acquired resistance to pesticides as well.

The reemergence of diseases such as diphtheria and whooping cough may be due to inadequate vaccination of the population. When the proportion of immune individuals in a population drops below a particular threshold, introduction of the pathogen into the population leads to an outbreak of the disease. In short, as we have seen with polio, we cannot be too vigilant or even too cautious in our fight against disease.

NEGLECTED DISEASES

Diseases are considered neglected when treatments either don't exist or are inadequate. Neglected diseases mainly affect people in developing countries, as in many countries of Africa and Asia. The term *most neglected* is used to mean diseases that occur among people who are so poor that there is no hope for purchasing treatments.

Why aren't more treatments available? Millions of people die each year of preventable and treatable diseases. Although cures exist, they were discovered in the industrialized Western world, mostly in the United States and Europe. They are therefore so expensive that most people in developing countries can't afford to get them. The costs are simply too high. When one month's prescription costs more than the entire family earns in a year, treatment becomes unattainable.

Human African trypanosomiasis, also called sleeping sickness, is a neglected disease. It is endemic in poor populations in remote rural areas of Africa. Left untreated, it is a fatal disease that now afflicts 500,000 people in Africa. Sleeping sickness is caused by a parasite carried by the tsetse fly that infects both humans and animals. The parasite multiplies in the bloodstream and lymph nodes, causing fever, weakness, sweating, and joint pains. Over time, it affects the brain, causing seizures, coma, and death.

Those infected may show signs of illness immediately or may not show any symptoms for years. However, they do become carriers of the disease, and whenever they are bitten by a tsetse fly, the insect picks up the parasite and spreads it to the next fly-bite victim. An estimated 60 million people in Africa are exposed to the infective bite of the tsetse fly. Animals like cattle can also become infected.

In 1960, the disease was brought close to elimination. But then it resurged dramatically as health systems broke down and control programs were abandoned or weakened by political problems and wars in Africa. Major epidemics are currently underway in central Africa in the countries of Angola, Congo, Uganda, Democratic Republic of Congo, Sudan, Ethiopia, Malawi, and Tanzania. Death in certain villages may reach levels as high as 50 percent of all residents. Infected individuals, having no access to health services, die in their villages due to the unavailability

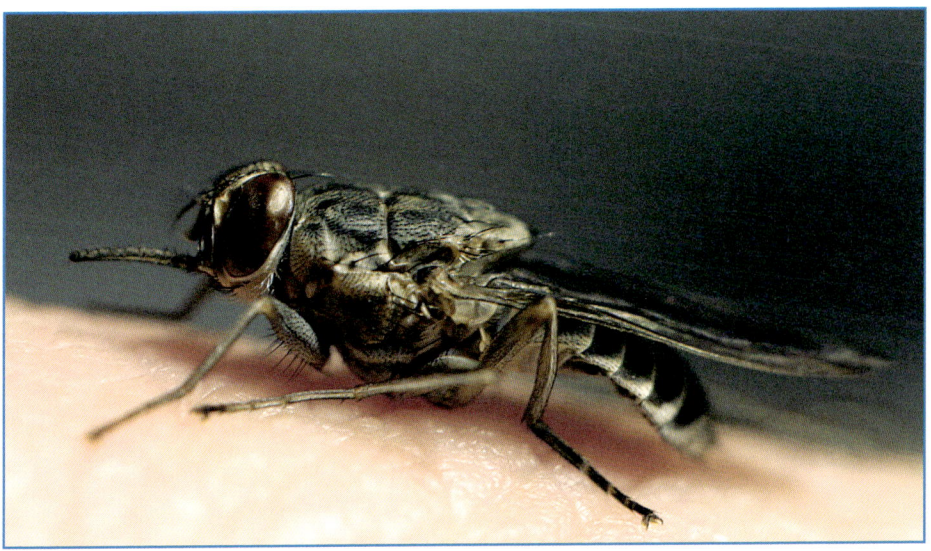

The tsetse fly is among the most harmful pests of sub-Saharan Africa, spreading sleeping sickness and other diseases. Sleeping sickness is a neglected disease that is curable but continues to wipe out much of the population.

of care. The cases reported each year are only a small fraction of the real number of infected individuals.

Sleeping sickness is a curable disease. Attempts to cure patients in the late stages have been partially successful with use of a highly painful and dangerous drug, Melarsoprol, developed during the 1940s. The drug, although available in small quantities, causes death among approximately 15 to 20 percent of those treated.

It has been known, however, by pharmaceutical companies for more than 10 years that eflornithine is a virtual miracle cure for sleeping sickness. In 1995, the drug was no longer manufactured due to high production costs, low profits, and its negative effect on cancer, for which it was originally being tested. But in 2001, the active ingredient reappeared in a women's vanity product called Vaniqua, intended to remove facial hair.

Sadly, because only poor people in poor countries suffer from sleeping sickness, there is no active research into new medicinal cures for the disease. So it remains a neglected disease.

GLOBALIZATION AND DISEASE

The risk of pandemic disease in this interconnected and fast-paced world continues to grow. The worldwide resurgence of dengue fever, the introduction of West Nile virus into New York City in 1999, the rapid spread of HIV in Russia, and the global spread of multidrug-resistant TB are examples of the effects of

CLIMATE CHANGE AND DISEASE

Climate change! The very words stir up a very heated debate. Some claim the world is getting warmer, others that it is actually getting cooler. What is indisputable however is that climate change is going to change the world as we know it. Malaria-carrying mosquitoes and deer ticks that spread Lyme disease are spreading and thriving in new places due to warming temperatures. This means that people who never had to worry about them will have to start. But mosquitoes and ticks are not the only health threats from global climate change. In fact, many experts claim that climate change is the biggest global health threat of the twenty-first century.

If global average temperature rises, we can expect more heat waves. The United Nations Intergovernmental Panel on Climate Change projects that Chicago will have 25 percent more heat waves by 2100. Similarly, the number of heat days in Los Angeles is expected to increase between four and eight times. These temperature changes will most severely affect people with heart problems and asthma, the elderly, the very young, and the homeless.

People who live within 60 miles (97 km) of a shoreline, or about one-third of the world's population, could be affected if sea levels rise globalization on the emergence and spread of infectious diseases. No nation is safe from the growing global threat that can be posed by an isolated outbreak of infectious diseases. Human pathogens can arrive rapidly anywhere in the world.

Globalization—increasingly integrated trade, economic development, human movement, and cultural exchange—is impacting patterns of emerging and reemerging diseases. Indeed, the emergence and spread of infectious diseases are the epitome of globalization. Never before have food, animals, commodities, and capital been transported so freely and quickly across political boundaries. Never before have pathogens had such ample

as expected over the coming decades, possibly more than 3 feet (1 meter) by 2100. Flooded homes and crops could make a billion people homeless. As it becomes hotter, the air can hold more moisture, helping certain disease carriers, such as the ticks that spread Lyme disease, thrive.

A changing climate could increase the risk of mosquito-borne diseases such as dengue fever, yellow fever, and viral encephalitis. Algae blooms in water could be more frequent, increasing the risk of diseases such as cholera. Respiratory problems may be aggravated by warming-induced increases in smog.

But will the climate change sufficiently to make all these apocalyptic predictions possible? Some experts claim that the so-called global warming is simply a normal part of the global climate cycle. In fact, some people even argue that rather than warming, the world is cooling, and this is nothing extraordinary. Who is right?

Regardless of the outcome of this debate, we need to be ready for new diseases and pandemic outbreaks. Globalization assures that the world we once knew is gone forever.

opportunity to hitch global rides on airplanes, people, and products. Infectious diseases are a threat to all nations, but especially for developing nations. As the HIV pandemic should have taught us, in the context of infectious diseases, no place in the world is remote and no person is disconnected.

Tourists travel the world. Millions of people are forcibly displaced by war. Migrant populations, especially refugees, are particularly vulnerable to infectious diseases. The emergence or resurgence of diseases such as multidrug-resistant TB has frequently been linked to the massive influx of immigrants from poor countries with higher prevalence of such diseases.

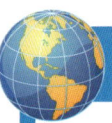

MAKING C◉NNECTI◉NS

HERE COME THE SUPERBUGS! ARE WE SAFE?

In 1943, penicillin was introduced as the "magic bullet" for curing many infectious diseases. By 1946, however, approximately 14 percent of *Staphylococcus aureus* strains isolated at a London hospital were resistant to penicillin. Today, scientists estimate that more than 95 percent of all *S. aureus* strains are penicillin-resistant.

After penicillin, additional antibiotics were rapidly isolated and developed, including streptomycin and the tetracyclines. Today, there are more than 100 antibiotics available. Nevertheless, some strains of at least three bacterial species, including TB, are resistant to all of these antibiotics. Health care workers fear the time is rapidly approaching when more deadly disease-causing organisms can resist all known antibiotics.

The invention of new and stronger antibiotic treatments has always been followed by new changes in bacteria as the bugs fight back, seeking to stay alive. Every time a person takes an antibiotic, bacteria that normally live in our bodies are killed. But some bacteria develop ways to stay alive and continue to grow and multiply.

The same advances in transportation technology that facilitate global travel by humans also allow rapid transcontinental movement of infectious disease vectors. For example, some researchers believe that the vehicle for introducing West Nile virus into the United States in 1999, the first occurrence of the disease in the Western Hemisphere, was an airplane carrying an infected mosquito. Mosquitoes can hitch rides in the wheel wells of airplanes. Moreover, global climate change may also produce geographic expansion of vector habitats.

The epidemiology of food-borne disease has changed significantly. Consumer demand and expectations have driven

Here is one simple and very common way that bacteria become resistant. If an antibiotic has been prescribed for 7 to 10 days, but you stop taking it when you feel better after three days, you have killed a large percentage of the bugs, but the ones that survive will develop a resistance to the antibiotic the next time they encounter it. This can lead to an increase in dangerous bacteria that are difficult to treat, resulting eventually in the superbugs we see today.

Misuse of antibiotics is the biggest reason for the emergence of superbugs. Decreasing antibiotic misuse is the best way to control resistance. Otherwise, we will have to keep outwitting the bugs with new antibiotics that they haven't seen before. This makes diseases more difficult and costlier to treat.

What measures do you, your family, your school, and your community take to prevent infections and maintain a germ-free environment? Can you think of a time when you or a family member was prescribed antibiotics unnecessarily? What effect do you think that had or could have had on the rest of your community?

food production and processing to become more geographically fragmented; foods produced in one area are processed elsewhere. The establishment of the World Trade Organization (WTO) has dramatically changed the ways in which all products, including food, are bought and sold.

Many countries do not have comprehensive food safety programs integrated into their public health strategies. Outbreaks of food-borne illnesses reveal the severe inadequacies of existing food safety regulations, even in developed countries. The free flow of food also raises serious concerns about the global spread of antibiotic resistance associated with the consumption of antibiotic-fed food animals.

Thus, the growing international market and increased human mobility have shaped and will continue to shape the global infectious disease landscape. Inability to monitor and provide adequate health care to the increasing numbers of internally displaced people or to monitor food-borne and trade-related infectious disease risk worldwide are compounded by the growing risk of bioterrorism. All of these have profound implications for global health.

This makes surveillance of mobile populations a new but necessary idea. The huge gap in TB rates between foreign-born and native-born U.S. residents is a good reminder. New standards and efforts are needed to monitor the health of mobile populations to reduce the risk of transmitting diseases to new areas.

Failing national public health programs also facilitate disease spread. For example, Russia is experiencing the emergence and reemergence of multiple infectious disease agents including hepatitis, HIV/AIDS, and TB as major epidemics. This is due to the tremendous economic, social, and public health fallout from the dissolution of the former Soviet Union. Unless public health efforts are taken seriously again, with some much-needed investments, global pandemics will win the war.

Drug resistance poses a major challenge worldwide. The serious problem of drug-resistant HIV infections in the United States

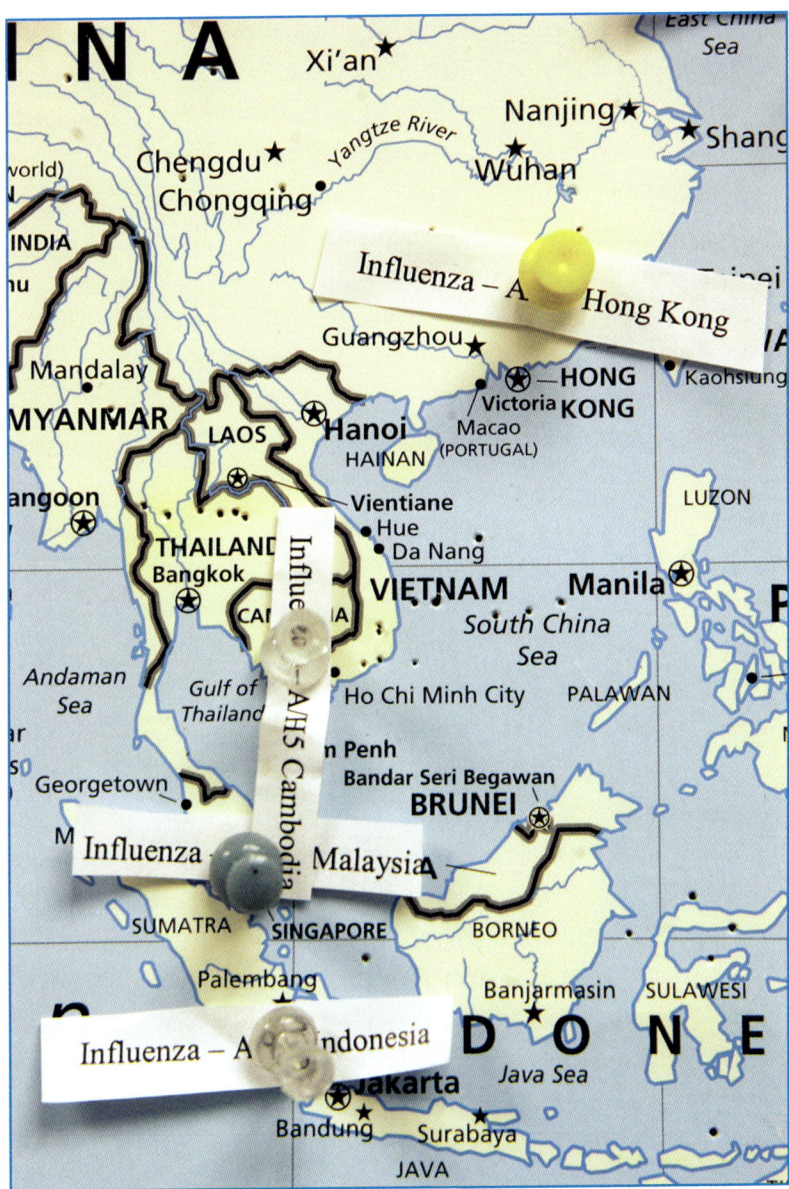

The U.S. Centers for Disease Control (CDC) mark influenza outbreak activity on a map to monitor activity and detect patterns. Increased human mobility and the global market have led to a proportionate increase in the spread of infectious disease. It is important for the global community to maintain health and sanitation standards.

suggests that improper use of new and powerful medications puts the whole world at risk. Vaccine effectiveness is severely limited by weak or nonexistent public health infrastructures and resource limitations. In developing countries, poor compliance with antibiotic regimens due to poverty also fuels drug resistance. As our ability to fight them decreases, superbugs become stronger and threaten us even more.

Weak global surveillance systems remain a major challenge. Many countries fail to report local disease outbreaks to avoid negative economic and political repercussions, such as trade sanctions and travel advisories. HIV threatens the viability of severely infected states. A rational approach to international control of communicable diseases is needed; it should be based on science, not political boundaries.

WHAT LIES AHEAD?

As this book comes to a close, there are three messages that need to be emphasized. First, global pandemics are here to stay. We need to get used to them and develop effective responses, including surveillance and treatment methods. Second, political boundaries provide no protection from disease outbreaks. Developed countries are as much at risk of disease outbreaks as are poor countries that are struggling with neglected diseases. Thus, a critical way to protect our own health is to help developing countries to improve their health care systems and solve their health problems. Finally, in matters of health and disease, geography matters. Where you live and work influence not only how long you will live, what diseases you will face, and how you will respond to them, but also when and how you die. In short, diseases don't need visas to travel and do not respect political boundaries, but where you live matters. Global cooperation is critical for our collective survival against infectious disease. There is no other alternative.

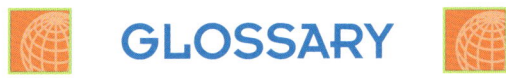

GLOSSARY

acute disease Sudden onset disease that has short duration, progresses rapidly, and needs urgent care. An acute myocardial infarction (heart attack) may last a week, but acute sore throat may last a day or two.

AIDS Acquired immunodeficiency syndrome. The final stage of infection with HIV, when the immune system CD4 cell count is less than 200/ml.

AIDS orphan A child who has lost either or both parents to HIV/AIDS.

asymptomatic polio Polio with minor symptoms including slight fever, headache, and sore throat, or no symptoms at all. Most people recover within 72 hours but may continue to pass the virus in their feces for weeks.

chronic disease An illness that a person has for a long time or an illness that goes away and keeps coming back. Diabetes is an example of a chronic disease.

communicable disease A disease that spreads from person to person.

degenerative disease A disease that results from deterioration of bodily function with old age. Cancer is an example of a degenerative disease.

drug resistance The ability of bacteria and other pathogens to withstand a drug that once killed them or slowed their growth. For example, TB that is resistant to the drug isoniazid is seen frequently. Previously, this was the drug of choice for treating TB.

emerging infectious disease An infectious disease whose incidence has increased in the past 20 years and threatens to increase in the near future. Includes diseases caused by newly identified pathogens or newly identified strains of known microorganisms.

endemic   Describes a disease that is always present in a community but usually at low levels. Malaria is endemic in most African countries, but epidemic outbreaks may occur.

epidemic   A sudden, severe outbreak of disease that affects more than the expected number of people in a community or region during a given time period.

HAART   Highly active antiretroviral therapy. Treatment with a very strong and powerful drug "cocktail," or combination, to suppress the growth of HIV, the virus that causes AIDS.

HIV   Human immunodeficiency virus. This is the virus that causes AIDS. It attacks the body's immune system, weakens it, and makes it difficult for the body to fight disease.

incidence   Number of new cases of a disease diagnosed within a time period, usually one year.

infant mortality rate   Number of children out of every 1,000 born who die before their first birthday.

inverse care law   Those who need health care the most have the least access to it. Poor people who usually have more medical needs also lack insurance or the means to obtain health care. People who live in an area with poor health care facilities usually have more health problems.

life expectancy   The number of years a person is expected to live based on statistics and probability.

multidrug resistance   The ability of a pathogen to resist multiple drugs that previously killed the bacteria or slowed its growth.

neglected diseases   Diseases for which treatments don't exist or are inadequate; pharmaceutical companies do not actively pursue new treatments for these diseases because they affect poor people or countries that can't afford to buy the medications or pay for the research. Trypanosomiasis is an example.

pandemic   An international disease outbreak; a sudden disease outbreak that becomes very widespread and affects whole world regions, continents, or the entire world.

paralytic polio Most severe form of polio, which attacks the central nervous system and may cause paralysis within hours. It occurs in about 2 percent of cases.

pathogen A disease-causing organism. It could be a virus, bacteria, or parasite. Influenza A (H1N1) is the pathogen that causes swine flu.

polio Poliomyelitis is an acute and sometimes devastating illness that may cause paralysis or death in about 5 percent of cases.

prevalence The total occurrence of a disease in a population. HIV/AIDS prevalence includes all living cases of the disease regardless of when they were diagnosed.

reservoir The site or population that harbors the disease-causing organism and thus serves as a potential source of disease outbreaks. For example, animals and insects such as the mosquito often serve as reservoirs for diseases that infect humans; similarly humans are the reservoir for the measles virus.

SARS Severe acute respiratory syndrome is an acute respiratory illness that is caused by a virus. Its symptoms include fever, dry cough, and breathing difficulties, often accompanied by headache and body aches. SARS became a global pandemic in 2003.

vertical transmission Transmission of a disease from mother to child usually during pregnancy or the birth process or after birth through breast milk during nursing.

XDR TB Extensively drug-resistant tuberculosis; relatively rare type of multidrug-resistant tuberculosis. It is resistant to almost all drugs used to treat TB. The remaining treatment options are much less effective and usually have more serious side effects and worse treatment outcomes. Such patients are more likely to die.

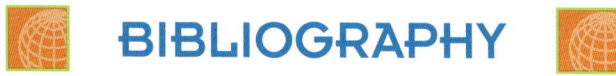

BIBLIOGRAPHY

Asiedu, Kingsley, R. Scherpbier, and M. Raviglione, eds. *Buruli Ulcer: Mycobacterium Ulcerans Infection*. Geneva, Switzerland: World Health Organization, 2000.

Centers for Disease Control and Prevention. *HIV/AIDS Surveillance Report 2007*. Vol. 19. Available online. http://www.cdc.gov/hiv/topics/surveillance/resources/reports/2007report/default.htm

Centers for Disease Control and Prevention. "Trends in Tuberculosis Incidence—United States, 2006." *MMWR Weekly*, March 23, 2007. Available online. http://www.cdc.gov/mmwr/preview/mmwrhtml/mm5611a2.htm.

Centers for Disease Control and Prevention. "2009 H1N1 Flu ("Swine Flu") and You." Available online. http://www.cdc.gov/H1N1flu/qa.htm.

Farrell, Jeanette. *Invisible Enemies: Stories of Infectious Disease*, 2nd edition. New York: Farrar, Straus, and Giroux, 2005.

Meade, Melinda, and Robert J. Earickson. *Medical Geography*, 2nd edition. New York: Guilford, 2005.

National Institute of Environmental Health Sciences. "Obesity and the Environment." Available online. http://www.niehs.nih.gov/health/docs/obesity-fs.pdf

Oppong, Joseph R. "Medical Geography" in *Geography of Sub-Saharan Africa*. Samuel Aryeetey Attoh, ed. Upper Saddle River, N.J.: Pearson, 2010.

UNAIDS. 2009. *2008 UNAIDS Annual Report: Towards Universal Access*. Available online. http://data.unaids.org/pub/Report/2009/jc1736_2008_annual_report_en.pdf

World Health Organization. *The World Health Report*. 2008. Available online. http://www.who.int/whr/en/index.html

FURTHER RESOURCES

Goldsmith, Connie. *Invisible Invaders: Dangerous Infectious Diseases*. Minneapolis: Twenty-first Century Books, 2006.

Foley, Ronan. *World Health: The Impact on Our Lives*. Austin, Texas: Raintree Steck-Vaughn, 2003.

Friedlander, Mark P. *Outbreak: Disease Detectives at Work*. Minneapolis: Lerner Publishing, 2009.

Hinds, Maurene J. *Fighting the AIDS and HIV Epidemic: A Global Battle*. Berkeley Heights, N.J.: Enslow, 2007.

Monroe, Judy. *Influenza and Other Viruses: Perspectives on Disease and Illnes*s. Mankato, Minn.: Life Matters, 2001.

Prentzas, G.S. *The World Health Organization*. New York: Chelsea House, 2009.

Weinman, Sarah. *Pandemics: Epidemics in a Shrinking World*. New York: The Rosen Publishing Group, 2007.

WEB SITES

www.kidshealth.org
This Web site provides useful, accurate, and current health information for children, teens, and their parents. It answers many questions on healthy growth and development, including sexual health. It includes in-depth articles, animations, and games.

www.kfwh.org
Kids for World Health. WHO-supported organization for kids helping to fight neglected diseases. Provides useful information about global health issues.

http://www.childrenshealthfund.org/publications/health-ed
Children's Health Fund (CHF) provides low-literacy health education materials to assist children and their families in learning about a variety of health-related topics.

http://northvalley.net/kids/health.shtml

Kids World Health and Medicine Links for Kids. Provides links to many Web sites dealing with health issues for children from a global and national perspective.

http://www.bam.gov/

Excellent Web site of the U.S. Centers for Disease Control and Prevention for kids. Body and mind (bam) teaches kids about fitness, food and nutrition, exercise, disease, and safety. Take a quiz, play a game, or create a fitness calendar.

http://kids.niehs.nih.gov/

National Institute of Environmental Health Sciences Kids Pages. Provides games, music, and other activities that introduce children to the impact of the environment on health. Encourages children to pursue careers in health, science, and the environment.

http://www.niehs.nih.gov/health/scied/index.cfm

The Environmental Health Science Education Web site provides educators, students, and scientists with easy access to reliable tools, resources and classroom materials.

PICTURE CREDITS

Page

12: Hillery Smith Garrison/ AP Images

16: Anat Givon/AP Images

20: Mohamed Sheikh Nor/ AP Images

27: Daniel Patmore/ AP Images

36: ©AFP/Getty Images

45: Denis Farrell/AP Images

49: ©REUTERS/POOL New

50: ©Infobase Publishing

56: ©REUTERS/STR New

59: Darron Cummings/ AP Images

65: Aijaz Rahi/AP Images

71: ©Getty Images

87: Guillermo Gutlerrez/ AP Images

89: Robert Mecea/ AP Images

99: Anton Fric/ AP Images

105: Charles Rex Arbogas/ AP Images

INDEX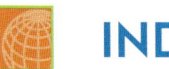

A

Aborigine people, 94
acute diseases, defined, 32
Afghanistan, 74
Africa
    HIV/AIDS in, 39–40, 43
    polio in, 65–66, 68–69
    reasons for severity of HIV/
        AIDS in, 44–46
    tuberculosis and, 57
aging, 37
agriculture, intensification of, 15
Ahmed, Aminu, 69–70
AIDS. *See* HIV/AIDS
airlines diversions, 88
Alice (in Zambia), 50
Amal (in Darfur), 45–46
Angola, 66
anthrax, 12, 37, 38
antibiotic resistance. *See* Drug
  resistance
antibiotics, 15, 38, 102–103
Antoninus, Plague of, 14
Aporkalypse, 87
aquatic insects, 35
Argentina, 90–91
Asma (in Pakistan), 76–77
asymptomatic polio, 64
Australia, 94
avian influenza (H5N1), 80, 81–84

B

Balochistan Boy Scouts
  Association, 77–78
Benin, 35
bicycle campaign, 77–78
Bill and Melinda Gates
  Foundation, 63, 70, 73
bioterrorism, 12
bird flu, 80, 81–84
Black Death, 14
Blakely, Georgia, 26
blood transfusions, 42

Bloomberg, Michael, 88
Bordet, Jules, 38
Botswana, 40
BSE (bovine spongiform
    encephalopathy), 12
bubonic plague, 14
Buruli ulcer, 33–35

C

Canada, 19, 80–81
CD4 cells, 43
Chad, 66, 67
chickens, 82, 93–94
children, 46–48, 48–50
Chile, 91
China, 57, 58, 79, 80, 82
cholera, 11, 13, 14, 22–23, 30
chronic diseases, defined, 32
climate change, 100–101
colds, 32
conflicts, 13, 16, 44–45, 67, 74–75
contagiousness, defined, 33
contamination, 12
cooperation, importance of, 17,
   63
cowpox, 38
crowding, 15
cultural beliefs, 44–45, 74–75

D

Darfur, 45
degenerative diseases, defined,
   37
dengue fever, 100
diabetes, 30, 32
diphtheria, 97
direct contact, defined, 34–35
directly observed therapy (DOT),
   54, 60
dosages, 47, 54
DOT. *See* Directly observed
  therapy
drinking water, 13, 22, 35, 84

drug resistance
    causes of, 15, 102–103
    malaria and, 29
    overview of, 104–106
    reemerging diseases and, 11
    tuberculosis and, 54
drugs, pediatric, 46–48
drug use, intravenous, 42, 58

E
ebola, 33
economics, 15. *See also* Poverty
education, 50
eflornithine, 99
Egypt, 79, 82, 91–94
emerging diseases, 10, 96–97
endemic diseases, defined, 29
environmental modification, 35
epidemics, 29–32
extensively drug-resistant
    tuberculosis (XDR TB), 54, 55, 111

F
farming practices, 15
FATA (Federally Administered
    Tribal Areas), 77
FDC (fixed dose combination)
    antiretroviral pills, 46–47
Fleming, Alexander, 38
flu. *See* Influenza
food supplies, 12, 24, 25, 35,
    103–104
freezers, 67, 69

G
Gates Foundation, 63, 70, 73
gender, 75
Gengou, Octave, 38
geography, health, 21–26
George (swine flu patient), 89–90
germ theory of disease, 37
Gilani, Yousuf Raza, 77
globalization, 10–12, 15, 24, 95,
    100–106
Global Polio Eradication Initiative,
    64–65
gonorrhea, 38
governance, 22–23, 67–68

H
H1N1 virus. *See* Swine flu
H5N1 virus. *See* Avian influenza
HAART (highly active
    antiretroviral therapy), 43–44,
    46, 50
health geography, 21–26
heart disease, 32
helper cells, 43
Hernandez, Edgar, 84–85
herpes, 36
highly active antiretroviral therapy.
    See HAART
history of medicine, 37–38
HIV/AIDS
    orphans and, 48–50
    overview of, 39–42
    as pandemic, 31
    Pascal's story (Kenya) and,
        46–48
    severity of in Africa, 44–46
    symptoms of, 42–44
    tuberculosis and, 54, 60
    in United States, 50–52
    vertical transmission of,
        35–36
homelessness, 58
homosexuality, 52
Hong Kong, 80, 93
horizontal transmission, defined,
    35
humor, 86–88
hunter-gatherers, 14

I
illiteracy, 67
immigrants, tuberculosis and, 58,
    102
immune system, 42–43, 54
incidence, defined, 32
India, 57, 71–74
indirect contact, defined, 35–36
Indonesia, 57, 82
infections, defined, 32–33
infectious diseases, defined, 32
influenza, 14. *See also* Avian flu;
    Swine flu
insects, aquatic, 35

Intergovernmental Panel on
  Climate Change (IPCC), 100
international trade, 104
internet, 15
IPCC. *See* Intergovernmental Panel
  on Climate Change
Iraq, 13
Islamic culture, 44–45, 75

J
Japan, 58
Jenner, Edward, 38, 73

K
Kano State Polio Victims
  Association, 69–70
Kent State University, 25
Kenya, 46–48
Koch, Robert, 37, 38

L
latent infections, 53
Lesotho, 40
life expectancy, 14, 18–19
Lyme disease, 100

M
mad cow disease, 12
malaria, 29, 97, 100
masks, surgical, 85
MDR TB. *See* Multidrug-resistant
  tuberculosis
Mecca, 68
Melarsoprol, 99
Mexico, 79, 84–90
microscopes, 38
migration, 102
milk, 41
minorities, 57–58
mosquitoes, 100, 101, 103
most neglected diseases,
  97–98
Mozambique, 40
Mugabe, Robert, 22–23
multidrug-resistant tuberculosis
  (MDR TB), 54, 102
mummies, 14
Muslims, 44–45, 68, 75

mutations, 11
mycobacteria, 33–35

N
Namibia, 40
Nasra (in Pakistan), 78
neglected diseases, 97–100
Neisser, Albert, 38
New York School for Autistic
  Children, 88
Nigeria, 57, 65, 66–69
1918 influenza, 14
nomads, 78
nursing, 41

O
Obasanjo, Olusegun, 68
obesity, 30–31, 32
oral polio vaccine (OPV)
  campaign, 64–65
organ donors, 42
orphans, 48–50

P
Pakistan, 74–78
pandemics, 31–32, 81–82
paralytic polio, 64
Pascal (AIDS patient in Kenya),
  46–48
Pasteur, Louis, 38
pathogens, defined, 32–33
peanuts, 26–28
penicillin, 38, 102
Peru, 14
pigs, swine flu and, 79, 91–94
pilgrims, 68
Plague of Antoninus, 14
plagues, 14–15, 38
polio
  Aminu Ahmed and, 69–70
  conflicts and, 16
  global eradication of, 70–71
  in India, 71–74
  in Nigeria, 65, 66, 68–69
  overview of, 62–63
  in Pakistan, 74–78
  reasons for spread and
    persistence of, 67–68

signs and symptoms of, 63–66
virulence of, 33
Polio Action Plan, 77
polio bicycle campaign, 77–78
Postal Service, 12
poverty
HIV/AIDS and, 44–46, 49–50
impacts of, 16–17
life expectancy and, 19
most neglected diseases and,
97–98
polio and, 69
tuberculosis and, 59–60
pregnancy, 41, 44–46
prevalence, defined, 32
prison, 58–59
public transportation, 47

Q
quarantine, 79

R
rape, 44–46
Reed, Walter, 37
reemerging diseases, 10–11, 97, 104
refrigeration, 67, 69
refugees, 16, 102
refusals, 76
relapsing fevers, 15
reservoirs, 16, 33–34, 60–61
resistance. *See* Drug resistance
Rome, 14
Russia, 104
Rwanda, 22

S
salmonella, 25, 26–28
sanitation, 13, 22, 35, 64, 72–74
SARS (severe acute respiratory
syndrome), 12, 15, 80–81
Saudi Arabia, 68
scale, 22–26
schools, 85
severe acute respiratory syndrome.
See SARS
sexual contact, 40–41, 42, 44–46
Shakila (in Pakistan), 78
Shibasaburo, Kitasato, 38

skin-eating bacteria, 33–35
sleeping sickness, 98–99
smallpox, 14–15, 38, 72–73
soap operas, 86
soil as reservoir, 33
Somalia, 73
South Africa, 40, 57
Speaker, Andrew, 55–57
spread, 10, 34–37
Staphylococcus aureus, 102
Strategic National Stockpile, 91
Sudan, 66, 67
superbugs, 102–103
surveillance, 104, 106
Swaziland, 40
swine flu (H1N1)
Argentina and, 90–91
Australia and, 94
Egypt and, 79, 91–94
future food needs and, 95
Mexico and, 86–88
origins of, 85–86
overview of, 84–85
as pandemic, 31–32, 79
United Kingdom and, 94–95
United States and, 88–90
syphilis, 14

T
Tamiflu, 91
T cells, 43
television, 86
terrorism, 12
ticks, 100
tomatoes, 25
tourism, 102
transfusions, 42
transportation, 10, 15, 47, 102–103
trypanosomiasis, 98–99
tsetse flies, 98
T-shirts, 87–88
tuberculosis (TB)
extensively drug-resistant, 54,
55, 111
international scare in 2007,
55–57
Koch and, 38
overview of, 53–54

in Peru, 14
reemergence of, 97
treatment of in rest of world,
    59–61
in United States, 57–59, 60
typhus, 15

U

Uganda, 34
ulcers, 33–35
UNICEF, 76–77
United Kingdom, 94–95
Urbani, Carlo, 80
urbanization, 15
vaccinations
    for avian influenza, 83–84
    development of, 38
    for polio, 62, 64–65, 67–69,
        72–73, 74–78
    refusal of, 76
    for smallpox, 73

V

Vaniqua, 99
vertical transmission, 35–36, 41
Vietnam, 58, 82

virulence, defined, 33
viruses, 37–38. *See also* Avian flu;
    HIV/AIDS; Polio; Swine flu

W

wars, 13, 16, 44–45, 67, 74–75
water supplies, 13, 22, 35, 84
West Nile virus, 100, 103
whooping cough, 38, 97
wildlife, 33
World Trade Organization (WTO),
    104

X

XDR TB. *See* Extensively drug-
    resistant tuberculosis

Y

yellow fever, 15, 37
Yersin, Alexandre, 38

Z

Zaire, 22
Zambia, 40, 48–50
Zimbabwe, 22–23, 30, 40

ABOUT THE AUTHOR

JOSEPH R. OPPONG is Professor of Geography at the University of North Texas in Denton, Texas. He has been teaching and conducting research at the university level for about 20 years. He enjoys travel, photography, writing and mentoring students. A native of Ghana, Dr. Oppong's research focuses on the geography of diseases and health services. His most recent research focuses on the geography of HIV/AIDS and tuberculosis in Texas and in Africa. He has published extensively on these topics. Dr. Oppong has served as Chair to the Medical Geography Specialty Group and also the Africa Specialty Group of the Association of American Geographers. He has taught Medical Geography and Geography of Sub-Saharan Africa for about 20 years.

 # ABOUT THE EDITOR

CHARLES F. GRITZNER holds the title of distinguished professor of geography at South Dakota State University in Brookings. He is now in his fifth decade of college teaching and research. In addition to teaching, he enjoys travel, writing, working with teachers, and sharing his love for geography with young people. As a senior consulting editor and frequent author for Chelsea House Publishers' MODERN WORLD NATIONS, MODERN WORLD CULTURES, EXTREME ENVIRONMENTS, and GLOBAL CONNECTIONS series, he has a wonderful opportunity to combine each of these "hobbies." Dr. Gritzner has served as both president and executive director of the National Council for Geographic Education and has received the council's highest honor, the George J. Miller Award for distinguished service to geographic education, as well as other honors from the NCGE, the Association of American Geographers, and other organizations.